Contents

* See footnote p. 90

List of Inserts

Acknowledgements

During the course of this project I benefited from the advice and encouragement of Hugh Burkhardt, Bob Lindsay and many others at Nottingham University, especially George Brown. I much appreciate all the time Judith Rowlands gave to typing and checking the script.

My thanks go, too, to Paddy Riley, David Wishart and Jane Restorick for piloting me through the fields of statistics; to Peter Haywood, Wendy Watts and Janet Mawby who provided patient guidance through the libraries; to Larry Reynolds who helped with the arduous task of the marking of the tests.

My greatest debts of gratitude, however, are to Freddie, without whose help the project could never have been undertaken, and to Lorna, Clare, Anna and Andrew for providing the essential support at home.

Finally I wish to acknowledge the permission granted by Baillière Tindall to print in Appendix D an extract from the booklets now published under the title, "Maths for Nursing".

Preface

Some years ago a teacher of nursing commenting on mathematical skills needed by nurses in doing administration said 'This is where my teaching has to be 100% successful. Very few teachers have to set themselves so high an objective'.

Yet very few teachers of nursing are 100% successful in teaching mathematical skills. Dr. Pirie has made a significant contribution to the safety of practice by analysing the mathematical skills needed in nursing, the level of competence needed and the difficulties associated in using those skills. Besides diagnosing difficulties, she has prescribed treatment and provided and tested tools for teaching mathematical skills.

Nurse students and nurse teachers will be grateful for the very clear and decisive prescription she has made and its contribution to effective teaching and safe practice. The study will be especially welcome in Schools of Nursing and it takes its place alongside studies from other disciplines which make a valuable contribution to nursing practice. Though technical, the work is immensely readable and I found my attention was held throughout.

McFarlane of Llandaff

Abstract

The basis for this research lies in the widely held view that nurses have severe difficulties in some of the mathematical areas essential to their work. There has been very little work done in this field and the aim was, therefore, to define these problem areas and then to go on to investigate ways of remedying the nurses' mathematical deficiencies. It is hoped that the findings generated will assist the training of future learner nurses.

The first stage of the research was to compile a taxonomy of the mathematical skills which are needed by a nurse, and to define the necessary mastery levels in these topics together with the upper bounds of difficulty which a nurse is likely to encounter during normal work.

Stage two was to discover the common problem areas within these topics. This was achieved by analysing data collected from learners using a specially designed mathematics test. Ways of anticipating the problems were explored.

Learners' awareness of their weaknesses was also investigated. The results of a self-assessment survey showed that learners were poor at assessing their own mathematical abilities. As a consequence of these findings a diagnostic test was devised.

The final phase of the research involved an experiment to indicate the most effective remediation treatment. Only methods which could be accommodated within existing training time-tables were considered. Comparisons were made between:

1. use of specially designed self-instructional materials;
2. externally motivated use of text-books;
3. self-motivated use of existing resources.

Each treatment was preceded by a diagnostic test with feedback to the learners.

Analysis of the results of the experiment led to three major conclusions.

1. In every topic the booklets were significantly more effective than any other treatment.
2. The reading list had no impact on the numbers achieving mastery and little on the general attainment levels.
3. Merely making learners aware of their weaknesses was not sufficient for any significant learning to take place.

The implications of these findings are discussed and some areas requiring further research are identified.

CHAPTER 1

Introduction

1. Context

The traditional image of the nurse as a girl with a vocation to tend the sick is no longer sufficient to ensure the optimum conditions for patient care in today's hospitals.

The ability to listen, and understand a patient's fears, to counsel, and care for the patient's physical condition is still vital. No less important, however, is the need for communication skills which will enable the nurse to receive and report, concisely and accurately, information on disease and treatment; information which is frequently of a scientific nature. The entry requirements for students of a good pass at O-level English (or Welsh) language, literature or history is intended to ensure a certain level of literacy among those who aspire to nurse.

Modern drugs and technology also place an increasing need for mathematical skills on those now entering the profession and this is not universally recognised, nor is the relevant expertise sought. Professor Perlstein, in 1979, commented:

> "It would be reasonable to suggest that those of us responsible for the education of health care professionals be critical of the assumption that students are well-endowed with arithmetic skills and add to our curriculums whatever remedial help we can offer to make drug administration more realistic and safe."

Drug administration is, however, not the only area of mathematical activity in nursing, and before effective remediation can be offered to learner nurses the necessary skills must be defined. While much recent research has been conducted into the needs of entrants to industry, little has been done within the Health Service. This in no way indicates a lack of concern over nursing errors, as the literature shows (Chapter 2), but rather an understandable deficiency in skill-definition and specialised mathematics teaching techniques among nurse tutors.

One specific example of the changing needs within the profession arises from the total commitment of the Health Service to S.I. units within a country still largely working with Imperial measurements. This has introduced problems of conversions, for communication with patients, and lowered awareness of error, for learner and tutor alike, when handling unfamiliar units. This comes at a time when powerful new drugs, with toxic levels close to the therapeutic dose, demand an increased need for accuracy in administration. In many cases, experience can no longer supply applicable safety checks and mathematical competence becomes paramount.

2. Rationale

The intention of this research has been to generate findings of relevance to Schools of Nursing when considering the mathematical abilities of the learners. The aim was to attempt to answer four questions:

1. What mathematical skills are needed by a nurse?
2. Which of these mathematical fields cause the most common areas of difficulty?
3. Are learners aware of their weaknesses?
4. How can remedial help best be given?

1. *The Mathematical Skills.* This question occasioned the need to produce an authoritative taxonomy of the required skills, since, although subjective lists were proposed by many tutors and nurses, no systematically researched inventory existed. An important constraint was imposed at this point: only that mathematics actually used on the job was to be considered.

2. *The Mathematical Difficulties.* The nature of a nurse's training is such that the time actually spent in the School of Nursing is short. Little profit would be had from attempting to teach all the mathematics which a nurse needs to know. It was, therefore, expedient to define those topics in which the majority of learners were experiencing problems, and concentrate the remediation in these areas.

3. *The Self-Assessment of Weaknesses.* Since not all of the learners were likely to need mathematical tuition, some form of selection was needed. If the participation in the remediation programme was to be by self-selection, then it was necessary to be sure that the learners knew their own mathematical weaknesses. Should their powers of self-assessment prove to be low, some other method of appraising them of their abilities and failings would have to be found.

4. *Remedial Help.* The opportunities for learning tend to fall into three categories: (a) group tuition, (b) externally motivated, individualised learning, (c) self-motivated learning from available resources. A second constraint was imposed at this stage: when investigating the effectiveness of the different remedial approaches, only those methods practicable within existing nurse-training programmes were to be considered.

Although this work considers only nurses in training, some of the findings also have clear implications for qualified staff, and these are considered briefly in the final Chapter.

3. Methodology

The research was partitioned into three sequential stages:

Stage 1 was to discover the mathematics encountered by nurses in their work and the levels of mastery needed. The observational and analytic techniques used to do this are set out in Chapter 3, together with the outcome.

Stage 2 was to design and administer a self-assessment task and mathematics test based on the topics defined in Stage 1 in order to elicit information on the nature and scale of the problem, and on nurses' cognizance of their own failings. The findings of this phase are given in Chapter 4.

Stage 3 was to consider ways of effecting remediation among learners. As a consequence of information gained in Stage 2, it was considered expedient to offer a diagnostic test to learners on entry to training, prior to commencing any remedial work. The writing of this test and the production of teaching materials are described in Chapter 5. Chapter 6 covers the design and performance of an experiment to test the success of various different remedial methods for learners in the introductory block of training. The results of this experiment are presented in Chapter 7. Relevant literature is reviewed in Chapter 2.

The final Chapter, 8, discusses the limitations of the research, some conclusions which may be drawn and the implications of the findings for Schools of Nursing and for nurses in general. Some indications for future investigation are also given.

4. Summary

The raison d'être of this study of nurses and their mathematics has been established at the beginning of this Chapter. The research has been defined as an attempt to answer four questions:

1. What maths do nurses use?
2. What maths causes them problems?
3. Are they aware of their problems?
4. How can they be helped?

The three stages of investigation have been outlined and references to the appropriate Chapters 3 to 7 given. The final Chapter offers some comments and suggestions on the basic problem of nurses and the mathematical skills they need.

CHAPTER 2

Review of Relevant Literature

Reported research in the field of nursing mathematics has been minimal, and this has had significant implications for the breadth and depth of this study. This review attempts to cover the related research into nurses' errors, specific learning problems and currently available teaching materials. Since self-instruction and self-assessment are both integral parts of the research, literature in these areas is also considered. The final sections of this Chapter are concerned with mastery learning and the measurement of change.

1. Nurses' Errors

Virtually no errors other than those of drug administration have been reported or investigated. In fact, most of the literature on nurses' errors is from the United States of America, since, although there is widespread concern over the mathematical abilities of nurses and learners in Britain, this does not seem to be backed up by funds for research or remediation.

Brown (1979), a risk management co-ordinator, reported a study in Michigan, which, while being primarily concerned with the cost of nursing errors, gives the following breakdown of mistakes in drug administration: wrong dose 20%; wrong drug 17%; omission 15%; wrong rate of infusion 13%; wrong route 11%; wrong time 11%; wrong patient and duplication of dose 13%.

Of these errors, wrong dose and rate of infusion, that is 33%, are likely to be mathematical errors. Apple (1976) reported only 10% of errors in dosage, while Barker and McConnell (1962) detected 21%. The reason for these discrepancies may well lie partially in the fact that only *detected* errors are counted—and both Newton and Newton (1977) and Barker and McConnell suggested that a very high proportion of errors go unnoticed. Under normal circumstances, the statistics can actually only be based on *reported* errors. Barker and McConnell in a special observational study (1962) recorded that of 51,200 observed medication errors only 36 were in fact reported by the nurse, and that this constituted 64% of the errors detected by the nurse. Both Birkhalter (1972) and Newton and Newton (1977) discussed the vital importance of reporting errors.

An alternative approach to error assessment is via simulation and testing. Williamson and White (1974) recorded that, in a programme designed to test the level of competence in pharmacology of practising nurses, one registered nurse out of 24 failed to reach the minimum acceptable level due "to a lack of competence in dosage calculation". Drug doses, however, are not the only area of nursing computation. An experiment to discover how accurately dried milk powder was measured out for infant feeds (Wilkinson *et al.*, 1973) showed 100% variation in one case and consistent over-concentration of powder in all cases. Clearly, there is great need for care in measurement and calculation connected with neonates and probably the most pertinent research conducted into drug computation errors was by Perlstein *et al.* (1979) with paediatric staff working in an intensive care unit:

> "New born drug doses are . . . related to weight, age and gestation" and "speed in performing the calculations" is a "requirement".

The method of testing was by simulated physician's orders. The results were horrific, but to a large degree have been confirmed by this present study. The mean percent error rate was 24·2% and:

> "56% of the errors tabulated would have resulted in administered doses 10 times greater or less than the ordered dose."

The nurses were asked to judge whether the doses they had calculated were appropriate for the infants specified:

> "In 59·2% of the problems . . . the nurses were unable to correctly decide if the dose calculated was appropriate."

Perlstein showed further that:

> "the percent correct scores did not correlate with years since graduation from training." In fact "the experienced nurse had a greater tendency to feel certain in making judgements (but) these judgements were frequently wrong."

Fatal drug dose errors are reported in the British press from time to time (Daily Express, 24.4.78, an error of units; Daily Telegraph, 22.4.81, an error of calculation; The Times 28.11.81, an error of decimal place value, to cite but a few) and the resultant enquiries may be reviewed in nursing journals (Hicks, 1981; Nursing Times, 1974; Nursing Mirror, 1974; among others). Some errors, due to unfamiliarity with the changing units, such as that over a dose orally prescribed as 'five minims', written in the notes as '5 mgm' and administered as '5 ml', (Nursing Times, 1974) are less likely to occur now that S.I. units are used throughout the Health Service.

Much was written in Britain at the time of unit changeover (Anderton and Bigg, 1972; Metrication Board, 1977; Baron, 1974; Lippert and Lehmann, 1978 for example), to inform the medical professions on S.I. units; unfortunately, many of the articles and pamphlets emphasised methods of conversion and were not aimed specifically at nurses. Jeffries (1978) and Watchorn (1976) both carried a chapter on S.I. units, and Glenn and McCaugherty (1981) have produced a comprehensive book for nurses on the new units. Perlstein *et al.* (1979) found, however, that:

> "far and away the most frequent computational error was associated with the misplacement of the decimal point,"

and this appears to be true, even in countries where decimalised units have long been in use (Tidskr Sver Sjukskot, 1976a and 1976b). Two such fatal incidents in 1981 alone are reported in the Medical Defence Union's Annual Report (1981).

In Britain, the Medico-Pharmaceutical Forum of the Royal Society of Medicine (1980) considered the kinds of drug dose errors likely, especially in the theatre. Errors where:

> "fractions of an adult dose have been prescribed for an infant but inaccurately calculated,"

are mentioned but the main emphasis is on communication and identification problems. The London Hospital reported an error rate of up to 15% in drug administration (Vere, 1965), corroborated by Aberdeen Royal Infirmary (Crooks *et al.*, 1965). Even outside the hospitals, Keywood (1978) makes a case for injections rather than oral medications to be administered by community nurses to improve the reliability of drug doses.

Many Hospital Boards in America have tried to bring greater safety to the wards by introducing the unit dose (Kern, 1968; Stewart *et al.*, 1976; Budd, 1971 for example) often simultaneously with primary nursing in place of team nursing (Walters *et al.*, 1979). The rationale of this system of drug dispensing is to shift the onus of calculation, transcription and charging to the pharmacist. Many hospitals reported (Palmer, 1980; Walters *et al.*, 1979; Batty in Canada, 1975) that contrary to expectations the time spent on drug administration did not decrease, and the omission rate rose. Perlstein *et al.*, (1979) pointed out that the increased delay in administration involved is not acceptable in intensive care wards, and Dexter and Applegate (1980) refuted the suggestion that "maths is becoming less important to nurses".

A few hospitals in Britain (Warwick, 1974; Leeds, 1973, for example) have also experimented with the unit dose system. Ford and Ellis (1973) discussed the additional problem that nurses felt they were prevented from using their judgement and initiative and this would result in an increased lack of skill in drug dose calculation and administration. Dexter and Applegate (1980) too, made this point. Other attempts at error reduction have rested on legibility of handwritten prescriptions and readability of standardised recording forms (Frost, 1972; Kenny, 1969; Scholes and Wigmore, 1967).

2. Remediation and Mathematical Needs

There are schools of nursing on both sides of the Atlantic where remedial mathematics has been attempted for learners but little information has appeared in the journals. In the United States Dexter and Applegate (1980) described one such project and much of their finding is substantiated by this present research. They verified that their students were having problems with mathematics and that test scores did, to a certain level, correlate with school grades, although learners were leaving school less well prepared than in the past.

There have been many articles discussing the implications for schools of the present mathematical needs of industry, (Hitch, 1978; Fitzgerald, 1976; Fitzgerald, 1978; Lindsay, 1980, etc.) and other employments (IMA, 1974–76; Howie, 1981; Fitzgerald, 1979) but only Cockcroft (1982) based on Pirie (1981) has covered nursing needs.

3. Existing Materials

A large number of published materials exist in the United States to enable nurses to learn mathematics. These fall into several categories:

a. those written for use as a class with tuition (Skelley, 1971; McClain, 1966; Lipsey, 1977; Ferster, 1973; etc)

b. those written solely with reference to drug doses (Weaver and Koehler, 1966; Carr and McElroy, 1976; Olsen *et al.*, 1978; Keane and Fletcher, 1980; Medici, 1980; Hart, 1981; etc.)

c. those written in a traditional 'text book' format, but intended for self-study (Price, 1963; Jessee and McHenry, 1975; Taylor, 1978; Dison, 1980; etc.) All of these have chapters on arithmetic (decimals, fractions, etc.) unrelated to nursing examples, before going on to drug dose calculations, often relying on algebraic methods, without any specific algebra teaching (Grostray, 1963; McElroy *et al.*, 1977; McHenry, 1980; etc.)

d. those covering the same ground as group c, but written as programmed instruction (Gilbert, 1973; Sackheim and Robins, 1974; Anderson and Vervoren, 1976; Saxton *et al.*, 1977; Eisenbach, 1977; etc.) or with stated objectives and pre- and post-test for each short section (Fitch *et al.*, 1977).

Unfortunately, all these American texts are largely irrelevant to the needs of British nurses since they place heavy emphasis on the use of fractions, and drug doses are worked in a mixture of apothecary, household and metric units. They have been briefly reviewed here since many nursing libraries contain copies of these books. In 1982 there were only five nationally published books written specifically for the British nurse: Rosier (1967) category a, Hull *et al.* (1977) category b, and Jefferies (1978), Watchorn (1976), Glenn and McCaugherty (1981) all category c. Several schools of nursing have, in addition, produced, for local use, materials for both class teaching and individual studies.

4. Special Learning Problems

Three factors affect particularly the mathematical abilities of learners entering nurse-training.

First, the nursing profession recruits girls in the ratio 7 : 1 to boys, and as Avent (1977) said:

> "Many are forced to specialise . . . at the age of 14. Girls, especially, drop mathematics in large numbers."

There is also much reported research to indicate that in adolescence girls are worse at mathematics than boys, (Badger, 1981), and it is mathematics, not merely arithmetic, which nurses need.

Second, there is the problem of limited transfer (Ausubel, 1968; Gage and Berliner, 1979) reported in the HM Inspector's report (Department of Education and Science, 1979, 1980). Indeed Slotnicke (1981) found evidence of it even among medical students and Hindam (1960), demonstrated the inability of students to cope with irrelevant information and unfamiliar technical terms in essentially simple mathematical situations.

The third factor derives from the unusual training situation in Britain where learners may be awarded a place in a school of nursing at 16 but be unable to take it up until 18. It is a profession, too, which attracts a large number of mature students. The result being that many learners have not come directly from school and may have suffered a considerable degree of forgetting (Slotnicke, 1981).

Even those who have remained in full-time education lose skills which they may not have practised significantly since primary school (Fitzgerald and Applegate, 1978). In fact Dexter (1980) found that there existed an inverse relationship between age and maths test scores among nursing learners.

A WHO paper in 1978 reported on a study into this problem and evidence for a test on entry is given by Ausubel (1968):

> "The most important single factor influencing learning is what the learner already knows. Ascertain this and teach him accordingly."

5. Self-instruction

Self-paced learning materials need not be confined to books, however, and both Wittkopf (1972) and Layton (1975) recommended a wide range of approaches within a module, to appeal to every student, including the use of hardware to provide audio and visual impact.

This type of instruction has various implications for the student. It places:

> "the responsibility for learning where it belongs—on the student" (Hindthorne, 1980)

and allows him:

> "to learn at a rate consistent with his abilities, background, and experience . . . without competition or pressure from peers" (Gentine, 1980).

Skarratt (1980) went so far as to recommend that nurse students:

> "must be encouraged to follow up topics which they find interesting, irrespective of the plan of training."

Hogstel (1976) questioned whether nursing students should in fact be allowed to proceed at their own pace since they need to acquire the skill of making:

> "decisions about patient care and they usually cannot make these decisions at their own rate of speed."

In contrast, Heath (1979) argued with reference to Open University experiences that the ability to make decisions and develop standards is more effectively achieved by student-centred methods. Lumsden (1974) issued a warning on the lack of evidence and research to show which programmes actually work and while discussing three nursing mathematics units produced at Sheffield, Marson (1975) wrote:

> "no attempts were made to compare programmed instruction with conventional methods of teaching; many experiments of this nature had been conducted in other fields and had not proved particularly fruitful."

Nonetheless, since then, Blatchley (1978) and Huckabay and Arndt (1976 and 1981) have both shown by controlled experiments that independent study projects do compare favourably with lecture-discussion type instruction. In a small pilot study Spencer (1979) went further and split the learners into four groups by academic qualifications. She reported that category A students (highest academic group) learned more effectively from self-teaching materials, while category D students benefited most from a formal lecture.

When considering tutors, Herman (1976) pointed out that in addition to enabling them to devote more time to individuals' problems it is a useful teaching method where every tutor is not "competent in every topic in a course". This can frequently be the case with mathematics in a school of nursing.

6. Self-assessment

Self-motivated use of these materials by learners depends upon self-awareness of an existing lack of skills. In 1980, Yunek developed a self-assessment form for nurses to complete, to assist themselves in determining their learning needs, and Nance (1969) felt that a group of Canadian nurses learned considerably from a self-grading exercise. No check was made, however, on the accuracy of their self-assessments. Cowen showed in 1975 that students were "wretchedly incompetent" at assessing their best and worst solutions in an examination. Morton and Macbeth (1977) and Burke (1969) agreed with this verdict, but offered opposing trends in self-assessment, with Morton giving evidence of students evaluating their learning significantly lower than their tutors and Burke stating that "self-ratings were always more favourable". In 1976, Huckabay and Arndt reported an experiment in which all the nursing learners overestimated the amount of knowledge they had before instruction. A second experiment in 1981 showed significant differences between self-assessed and tested scores but no significant correlation. Daines (1978) divided his students into two groups by academic ability and demonstrated that while the high achievers "were quite realistic in their expectations", the lower group significantly overestimated their abilities. In an earlier study, Russell (1953) determined that boys rated themselves lower than girls, with the highest intelligence group underestimating and the lowest group overestimating.

The inconsistency of the findings of research in this field gives credence to the recommendation of Jernigan (1980) and Huckabay that:

> "teachers (should) rely more on objective tests to measure the entering behaviour of the student than on subjective evaluation."

7. Libraries

An obvious learning resource not so far mentioned is the nursing library. Unfortunately:

> "evidence that the majority of nurses do not read professional literature is strong." (Fitton, 1980).

That:

> "nurse training still largely involves a highly didactic approach" (Tabor, 1979).

is given also by Lindsay (1980b) as the cause of the minimal use nurses make of libraries, although lack of facilities is also significant; out of 402 libraries in the Directory of Medical Libraries in the British Isles, only 29 give access to nurses (Lindsay, 1980a). Many schools of nursing, of course, have their own separate library facilities. Shanks (1979) suggested that many nurses:

> "feign disinterest to hide inadequacy" and "incompetency on the subject of retrieval of information."

It is certain that figures such as those produced by Fisher and Shrank in 1971—only 68% of nurses in a group of 13 hospitals had read a book on their sphere of work in the proceeding 12 months; only 38·5% claimed to have used the library—indicate that libraries are a little used learning resource. More recent information from a survey in Northern Ireland (Myco, 1980) revealed 70% of nursing officers and 90% of ward sisters have never used the library services available. The introduction of organised library utilisation courses is supported by tutors and librarians alike (Bond, 1980; Stephenson, 1978; Boorer, 1969; Walser, 1977).

8. Mastery Learning

In 1976, Pickup stated that:

> "in vocational exams . . . the answer is criterion-referenced testing, (with) a clear statement at the start of the course of the objectives . . . and what constitutes the absolute performance."

In the field of mathematics it is vital for nurses to "achieve a predetermined competency level" (Gentine, 1980). Norm-referenced testing has no place here, although the concept of mastery learning (Bloom, Hastings and Madus, 1971) does contain the inherent assessment problem of determining the test and score which indicates that mastery has been obtained. Block (1971) contended that 80% to 85% is a reasonable required score, and that insistence on scores higher than this is not merely unreasonable, but may even have a negative effect on motivation. Many educationalists would agree with the idea that a reasonable target for students would be to cover 90% of a course with 90% mastery, that is 81% mastery of complete course (Lawler, 1974; Harris and Ligvorl, 1974); some recommended lower levels of 75% (Emerson, 1975; Airasian, 1972). Keller, however, who designed the Keller Plan for learning, based on small learning units with sufficient time to reach set mastery levels, is quoted by Bent (1974) as saying at a conference in Rome in October 1972 that tutors should:

> "require mastery to perfection before allowing a student to take an exam on the next unit."

This is possibly too stringent a target for all courses, but:

> "there are times when the 90% or 100% learning requirement is appropriate. In courses where students are taught basic skills and knowledges which are critical to subsequent learning and/or life success, this mastery requirement is sensible." (Mueller, 1976).

The postulation by Carroll (1963) that a student will succeed given enough time, indicates that a self-instructional approach may be the optimal method of tuition in this context.

9. The Measurement of Change

The third stage of this investigation into nursing mathematics is concerned with the value of various treatments, judged in the context of a 'pre-test, treatment, post-test' experiment. A brief review of the extensive literature in this area is given here, but only as it relates to the present research.

Adequate guidance on the design of such experiments can be had from many sources including Campbell and Stanley (1967), Cook and Campbell (1979), Fisher (1951). Having performed the experiment, there exists the problem of measuring the change which has been effected.

The instinctive approach is to consider the gain between pre- and post-scores. This method was, however, condemned by Cronbach and Furby (1970), Lord (1967) and Linn and Slinde (1977) the major defects being the negative correlation of gain with pre-score—particularly in evidence where a natural ceiling exists, as in mastery testing—and the unreliability which can in fact be such that:

> "gain scores can appear to reflect learning that actually does not occur" (Stake (1971).

In contrast, Richards (1975), concluded that difference scores were:

> "as good as the more complicated methods" and had the added advantages of ease of computation and of being "more meaningful to non-researchers."

The generalisability of his conclusions, however, are restricted by the assumptions of his model.

The use of residual scores goes some way towards a better interpretation of change, but again low reliability must give rise to caution (Linn and Slinde, 1977). Cronbach and Furby (1970) suggested that a better estimate of true change may be had by considering further data relevant to the test subject, but these are often unavailable. The search for a 'true difference score' has led to the discussion of errors of measurement (Lord, 1967—in particular in linked observations; Linn and Slinde, 1977—multiple regression methods; in Cronbach and Furby, 1970; and use of control variables—Feldt, 1958). Cronbach and Furby argued, however, that:

> "gain scores are rarely useful, no matter how they may be adjusted or refined."

One of the major hurdles in educational research is the frequent lack of randomly assigned testing groups. Fisher (1951) discussed controlling pre-treatment differences and Feldt (1958) compared simple analysis of variance, analysis of covariance and analysis of variance of randomised differences as "techniques to improve the precision of experimental design". In 1967 and 1969 Lord exposed the paradox which can arise from use of analysis of covariance and concluded that there:

> "simply is no logical or statistical procedure that can be counted on to make proper allowances for uncontrolled pre-existing differences between groups."

Nevertheless, as Linn and Slinde (1977) pointed out:

> "many practical decisions must be made without the aid of randomised experiments."

Even when considering merely the achievement of mastery levels, Hambleton and Novick (1973) suggested that 'true' levels and scores be considered, and Novick *et al.* (1973) provided the theory for a Bayesian estimation procedure to calculate the error of the observed score. A simpler solution proposed by Cronbach and Furby is that, provided "the errors of measurement are random", the post-test is an "entirely suitable" variable with which to work.

10. Summary

In this Chapter, a wide range of literature has been reviewed as it relates to nursing mathematics. Reports of nursing errors, mainly from the United States, give the type and frequency of errors committed, and special attention has been paid to neonatal care, and the British problems due to the change to S.I. units. The value of the unit dose is discussed. Little has been published on remediation or nurses' mathematical needs, but three special learning problems affecting Schools of Nursing are presented. These are:

(i) that nurses are predominantly female and girls are worse at mathematics than boys
(ii) mathematics learned at school is not necessarily transferred to the nursing situation by learners
(iii) many entrants to nursing do not come directly from full-time education.

Existing teaching materials, mostly American, are reviewed and the merit of self-paced materials is considered. The results of research into the abilities of students to assess themselves accurately are inconsistent and recommendations for an entry-test are considered. Nursing libraries are exposed as a much under-used resource. Literature suggests that in vocational training, nurses should not be judged relative to the norm, but should achieve a pre-determined competency level, although there are difficulties involved in the selection of this mastery level.

Finally, references to work on experimental design are given and the controversy over the measurement of change is examined.

CHAPTER 3

Compiling the 'Maths for Nurses' Taxonomy

The first stage of the research was to identify the mathematical skills needed by nurses in their work. The procedures adopted and the taxonomy devised are set out in this Chapter.

1. Observation

The literature review did not reveal any previous attempts to define precisely what mathematics is used by nurses while working on the wards, and so reports of three job analysis projects (Scottish Home and Health Department (1967), Williams (1977), Moores and Moult (1979)) were used to compile an observation schedule in which the activities were categorised as (i) "unlikely to contain mathematical activity", (u); (ii) "possible mathematical activity", (p) or (iii) "definite mathematical activity", (d). The schedule was then checked against assessment papers for student and pupil clinical examinations to ensure that at least all assessed activities would be observed.

The aim was to identify as far as possible all those activities which on some occasion, although not necessarily always, contained an element of mathematical skill. The majority of observational schemes, developed for the classroom, but transferable to the ward, fall into one of four categories:

(i) Recording activities at regular time intervals (Polansky *et al.*, 1950—15 minutes; Cornell *et al.*, 1952—5 minutes; Flanders, 1970—3 seconds);
(ii) Checking against a pre-determined check-list for frequency (McGee, 1955; Wrightstone, 1951);
(iii) Unobtrusive, formal observation where communication between subjects and observer is discouraged (Small *et al.*, 1979; Conners and Eisenberg, 1966);
(iv) Case studies (Adelman and Walker, 1975; Emmerich, 1968).

None of these techniques was entirely appropriate to the project, however, and the author adopted the informal strategy of participation in the general ward activities and nurses were encouraged to discuss and indicate any tasks which they felt relevant. The schedule was to be used as a basis to ensure that every task was observed. Once the position of those tasks in category (i) ("unlikely") was confirmed they were deleted from the schedule and the remaining tasks were observed in a variety of wards over three months and the mathematical content analysed and recorded.

2. Informal Interviews and Examination Questions

Approximately 150 ward nurses were questioned informally about the tasks and three series of books (Bailey, 1980; Gillies and Alyn, 1968; Lewis and LuVerne Wolff, 1978) containing sample test questions were scrutinised for any mathematics implicitly required in order to pass the final examinations. It was important to keep in mind that the objectives at this stage were to list and analyse only mathematics required on the job. For this reason, topics, such as statistics were not included in the taxonomy being compiled, even though they occurred in recommended 'maths for nurses' textbooks.

3. Tutors' Comments

The mathematical topics having been ascertained, 18 School of Nursing tutors completed a detailed questionnaire (Appendix A) aimed at delineating the upper bounds of the mathematical skills needed. These answers were compared with the results of the observation analysis and the mathematics needed by a nurse was defined as 24 skills with certain specified upper bounds. This list with its bounds was sent to 35 nurse tutors for their comments. Thirty-one of these were returned and investigated, but it was not found necessary to make any changes in the taxonomy. Discrepancies and comments did occur over topics which the tutors thought unnecessary, but which had, in fact, been observed on the ward. This underlined the need for the lengthy task analysis method used, rather than the employment of the 'expert' method recommended by Lindsay *et al.* (1974).

4. The Taxonomy

The following four pages contain Insert 3.1, giving the list of skills needed (column 1), an indication of the upper level of difficulty that a nurse can expect to encounter in each case (column 2) and one fairly common example, usually out of many, of a practical task requiring

Insert 3.1: The 'Maths for Nurses' Taxonomy

TOPIC	UPPER BOUND (U) and MASTERY LEVEL (M)	USES (Common Examples)	BEHAVIOURAL OBJECTIVES To be able to—
A Addition of whole numbers	1204 + 359 (U, M)	Fluid balance chart—see Insert 3.2	add integers of up to 4 digits
B Subtraction of whole numbers	1320 − 575 (U, M)	Fluid balance chart—see Insert 3.2	subtract integers of up to 4 digits
C Multiplication of whole numbers	125 × 4184 (U, M)	Convert calories to joules (1 C = 4184 J) Weight related drugs, paediatric feeds, etc.	multiply integers of up to 4 digits
D Division with whole numbers	925 ÷ 125 (U, M)	Drug doses: 925 mg available as 125 mg/ml. (From 25 mg/kg, weight = 37 kg)	divide integers of up to 4 digits by integers 1–9 and multiples of 5
E Addition of fractions	$\frac{1}{2}+\frac{3}{8}$ (U, M)	Several injections of the same drug: Drug available as 1 mg in 5 ml. Mr X needs $\frac{2}{5}$ mg; Mr Y, $\frac{4}{5}$ mg; Mr Z, $\frac{3}{5}$ mg. Total $\frac{9}{5}$ mg = $1\frac{4}{5}$ mg $\Rightarrow$ need 2 × 5 ml ampoules	add fractions with simple or common denominators, recognising equivalence
F Multiplication of fractions	$1\frac{1}{2}\times\frac{3}{5}$ (U, M)	$7\frac{1}{2}$ units of 40 strength insulin $= 7\frac{1}{2}\times\frac{1}{40} = \frac{15}{2}\times\frac{1}{40}$ ml	multiply mixed fractions with simple denominators, recognising equivalence
G Addition of decimals	10·26 + 3·055 (U, M)	Total energy in diet = 41·84 J + 28·05 J. Paediatric feeds, expected weight gain, etc.	add decimals of up to 3 decimal places

H Subtraction of decimals	$4{\cdot}05 - 3{\cdot}965$ (U, M)	Weight gain of baby $= 4{\cdot}05$ kg $- 3{\cdot}96$ kg. Special diets	subtract decimals of up to 3 decimal places
I Multiplication of decimals	$0{\cdot}725 \times 1{\cdot}32$ (U) $0{\cdot}725 \times 132$ (M)	Drug dose 0·75 g, available 1 g in 0·5 ml. Dose $= 0{\cdot}75 \times 0{\cdot}5$ ml. Drug doses normally available as x mg per y ml where y is an integer	multiply a decimal by an integer with up to 3 figures
J Division of decimals	$26{\cdot}4 \div 75$ (U, M)	Drug dose 62·5 mg, available 25 mg in 1 ml dose $= \frac{62{\cdot}5}{25}$ ml	divide a decimal by the integer 1–9 and multiples of 5
K Division by decimals	$0{\cdot}45 \div 0{\cdot}6$ (U, M)	Drug dose 0·45 mg, available 0·6 mg in 1 ml dose $= \frac{0{\cdot}45}{0{\cdot}6}$ ml particularly paediatric work	divide a decimal by a single digit decimal
L Converting fractions to decimals	$\frac{5}{8} = (0{\cdot}625)$ (U, M)	Injection dose $= \frac{2}{5}$ ml $= 0{\cdot}4$ (Convert to use syringe)	understand that quantities commonly accepted as fractions still mean 'division' and are a simple case of D
M Converting decimals to fractions	$1{\cdot}25 = (1\frac{1}{4})$ (U, M)	Drug dose $= 1{\cdot}25 = 1\frac{1}{4}$ tablets	convert 'x.25', 'x.5', 'x.75' to fractions, where x is an integer
N Percentage	20% of 800 (U, M)	Solutions 2 litres of 10% Dextrose contain $\frac{10}{100} \times 2$ l dextrose Urine-sugar levels—percentage used as a label	calculate simple percentages

Insert 3.1: The 'Maths for Nurses' Taxonomy

TOPIC	UPPER BOUND (U) and MASTERY LEVEL (M)	USES (Common Examples)	BEHAVIOURAL OBJECTIVES To be able to—
O Ratio problems	x mg required of a solution 1 to 5 or a solution 2 mg {per / in} 3 ml (U, M)	Drug doses	calculate drug doses from a doctor's prescription
P Use of S.I. units	g, l, mol, m, J, Pa — mega, kilo, unit, milli, micro (U)	Convert 0·025 mg to micrograms	work accurately with the S.I. units most frequently encountered
	g, l, m, J — mega, kilo, unit, milli, micro (M)	All hospital measurements now in S.I. units, but Pascals and moles less frequently encountered than the others	
Q Using formulae	Word formulae of form $A = \frac{B+C(D+E)}{F}$ (U)	Expected weight = Birth weight + (Age in weeks − 2) in kg × normal weight gain in kg	calculate, using a formula expressed in words, infant feeds, fluid requirement, expected weight gains, drug doses, etc.
	Word formulae of type $\frac{A}{B} \times \frac{C}{D}$ or $A \times B + C \times D$ (M) and selection of values from extra data	Drug doses, food requirements etc. The more complex formulae occur in specialist departments	

R Use of tables	S.I./Imperial conversions (U, M) Age/Normal weight gain	Most frequently used for communication with patients: 55·25 kg = 8 stone $9\frac{1}{2}$ lb. Paediatric progress assessment	obtain information, convert S.I. ↔ Imperial units from printed tables
S Meaning of Indices	Understand the change between $a \times 10^y$ and $z \times 10^y$ and $z \times 10^p$ (U)	Path. Lab. report 'Red cell count $= 4{\cdot}5 \times 10^{12}$	understand scientific reports on patients; information usually given in standard form
	Meaning of $a \times 10^y$ (M)	The nurse is usually the first person to see the path. lab. reports and therefore carries the responsibility of alerting the doctor if necessary	
T Meaning of decimal place	0·1 > 0·07 (U, M)	Safety in estimation and accuracy in calculation. Known adult dose 0·05 mg implies child's dose of 0·25 mg has been miscalculated	know the meaning of digits in various decimal places
U Making and filling in tables	Intensive care $\frac{1}{4}$ hourly record (U, M)	See fluid balance chart Insert 3.2	record information in an appropriate printed table
V Plotting graphs	Multi-graph and Diabetic graph (U, M)	See illustration of temp, blood pressure, pulse, respiration. Also urine-sugar with $\frac{1}{4}\%$ etc. Insert 3.3	record information on a graph with scales already determined
W Interpreting graphs	Paediatric I.C. graph. Judge weight against a standard weight graph. (U, M)	Alert the doctor to significant change in temperature	read information off a graph and form judgements from these readings
X Addition of negative numbers	1·2 + −0·3 (U) (non-essential)	Combining lens strengths in eye out-patients department	add +ve and −ve simple decimals

Insert 3.2: Fluid Balance Chart

Paediatric Fluid Balance Chart

EACH CHART COMMENCES 0800 HOURS
ALL ENTRIES IN MILLILITRES
ALL INTRAVENOUS RECORDINGS IN RED

CHART No. 2 WARD F21 WEIGHT .... kg

DATE	INTAKE							OUTPUT				
	Intravenous Route				Oral/Other Route	Cumulative Total in		N/G Aspirate and Comments	E/P Urine	Lt Uts² re Tube/ Drain	Stools and Comments	Cumulative Total Out
TIME	Type/Fluid and Hourly Rate of Flow	Burette Reading	mls in last hr	Drug Vol	Type/Amount of Feed	IVI	Other					
0800		0/60	50			50	mls	10 mls Aspirate green fluid				10 mls
0900		15/60	45			95	mls	15 mls Aspirate green fluid N/G Tube removed				25 mls
1000	500 ml 0.18% Saline 4% Dextrose c̄ 50 mls hly	10/60	50		10 mls H_2O	145 ml	10					
1100		20/60	40		10 mls H_2O	180	20					
11.30									110 ml	5 mls		200 ml
1200		15/60	45		10 mls H_2O	230	30					
1300		15/60	45		10 mls H_2O	275						
1400		20/60	40		10 mls H_2O 50 mls orange	810	50 100					
1500		10/60	50		100 ml Orange	360	200			10 ml		210 ml
1600		10/60	50		40 ml c̄ orange	410	240					
1700		35/60	25		200 Blackcurrant	435	440					
1800		10/60	50	2.5 ml		487.5						
1900		IV Discontinued 0	60		100 mls Orange	547.5	540		400	250		860 ml

the particular skill (column 3). Nursing tasks and the associated skills required are discussed in depth in Pirie (1981), but a few relevant comments on the compilation and content of the taxonomy are given below.

1. After deliberation, it was decided to include "addition of negative numbers" in the topic list, because although a comparatively rarely used skill by most qualified nurses, it occurs in an area, namely eye outpatients, where a large number of learners do some of their training (Pirie, 1981).
2. Since the Health Department adopted the S.I. units and abandoned the use of the Imperial and Apothecary systems, the need to calculate with fractions has almost disappeared, although many tutors have not yet recognised this fact. Concurrently, of course, the need for accurate decimal handling has increased. In particular in the area of paediatric nursing, drug doses of say, 0·05 mg per kg of body weight, are not uncommon and precision both in the calculation and the administration is essential.
3. The advent of the pocket calculator has not eliminated the need for mental arithmetical skills, since there are many occasions in nursing when use of a calculator is inappropriate (Pirie, 1981). Even when using a calculator, the nurse should be able to judge whether the answer to her calculation is reasonable, basing her decision either on past experience or on mathematical estimation.
4. Medicine is an area where modern technology is creating dramatic and rapid changes in the skills which are required of all the associated professions. Use of computer technology has meant that although some nurses may no longer need to calculate and set up by eye a drip-rate for an infusion of x litres over y hours, others are required to recognise and react to specific wave patterns appearing on cardiac monitors. Clearly one cannot predict all the changes which will affect the nurse of the future, but a sound mathematical base is essential if she is to be able to respond to the new demands made upon her skills.
5. Recording and interpreting graphs is an important part of every nurse's work, and since the format of the standard graph forms vary between wards, nursing areas and even consultants, the nurse needs to be confident in her understanding of scale and plotting techniques. Insert 3.4 illustrates a lack of comprehension by a nurse of the visual impact intended to aid diagnosis.
6. There is one particular skill, which, although very important to a nurse, is not listed separately in the taxonomy because it is not definable and teachable as a specific mathematical topic. This is the ability to select from a profusion of details and numbers that information which is relevant to the calculation to be performed.

Insert 3.3: A Multi-Graph

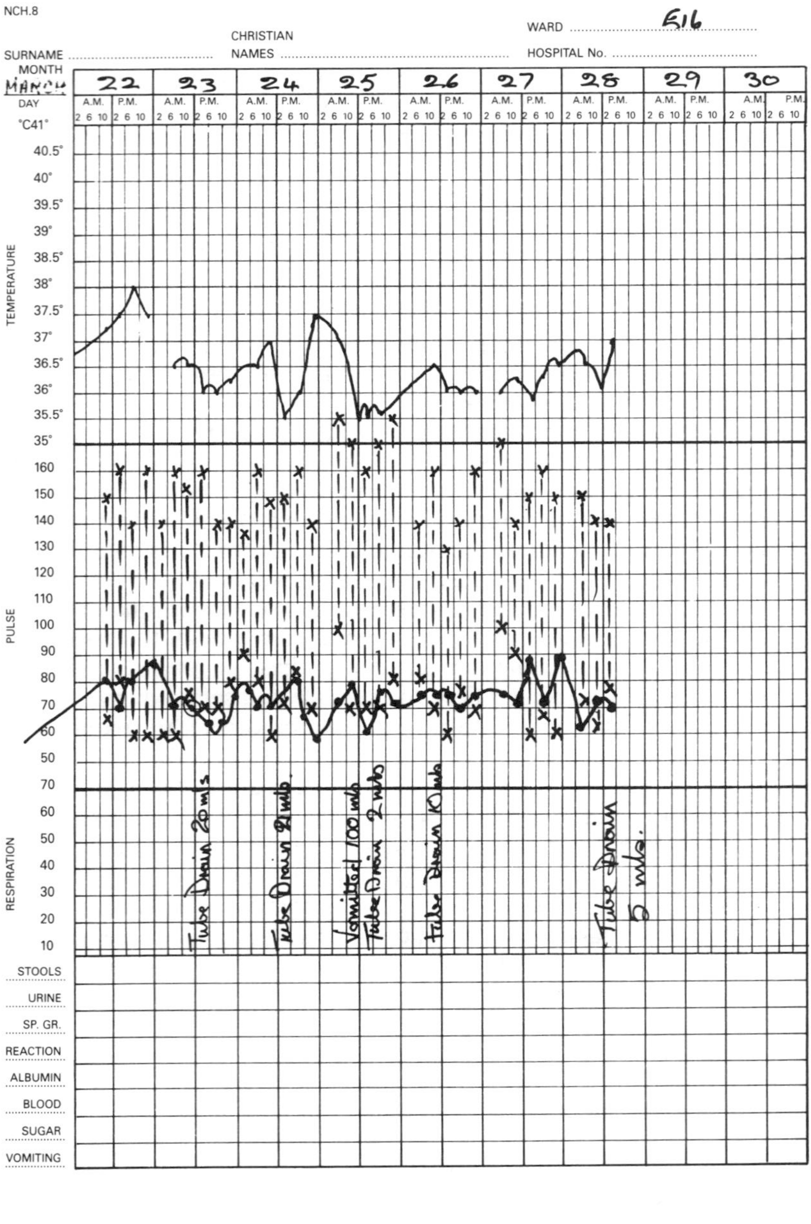

Insert 3.4: Diabetic Chart

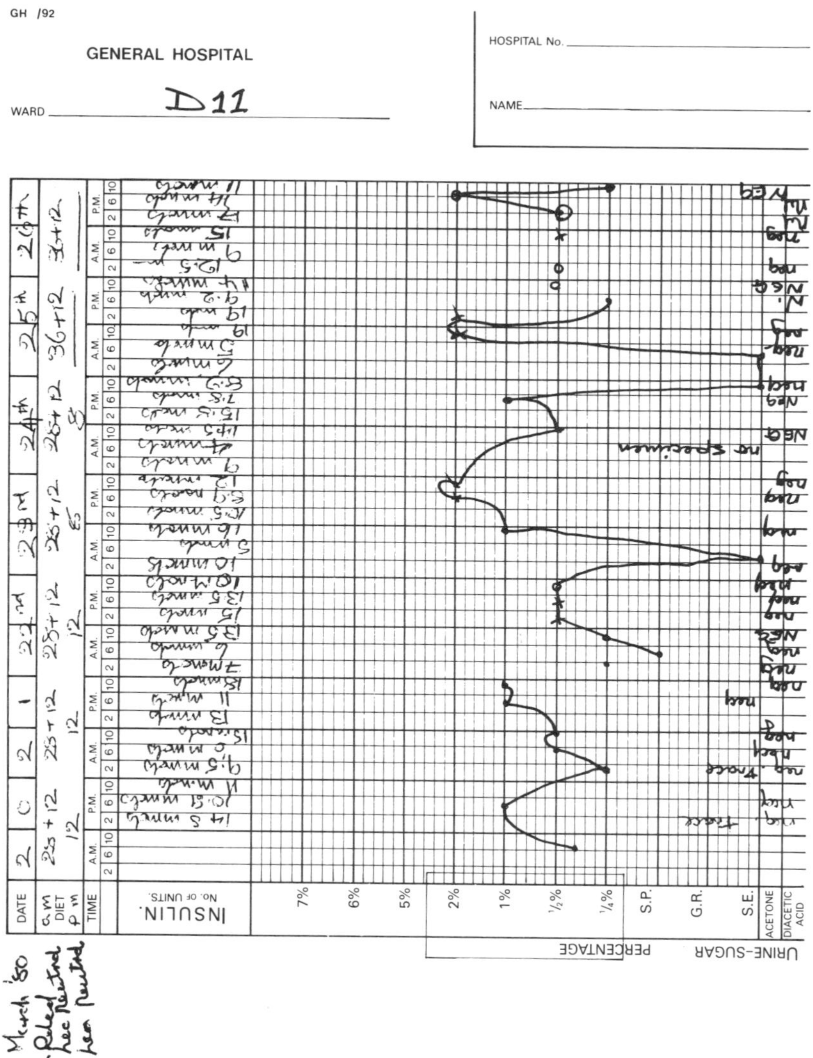

Some examples will be given to illustrate this point:

(a) A nurse needs to calculate drug doses for

(i) a 7 year old, weighing 22 kg (see record card) prescribed

$\frac{|0{\cdot}45 \text{ g atrophine sulphate}|}{\text{doctor's prescription}}$ available as

$\frac{|600 \text{ mg in 1 ml}|}{\text{ampoule label}}$

Here the 7 years and 22 kg are irrelevant.

(ii) a 6 year old weighing 17 kg, (see record card), prescribed

$\frac{|0{\cdot}5 \text{ mg/kg diazepam}|}{\text{doctor's prescription}}$ available as

$\frac{|10 \text{ mg in 2 ml}|}{\text{vial label}}$

Here, only the 6 years is irrelevant.

(b) A nurse needs to calculate the rate of drip for a prescription of "1000 mg drug in 500 ml of 5% dextrose in water over 6 hours", knowing the equipment delivers "60 microdrops per ml". Here 1000 mg and 5% are irrelevant in calculating the rate of drip.

(c) A prescription for a patient weight 54 kg, height 1·8 m, with leukaemia is for "72 mg/m^2 (body surface area) of doxorubicin hydrochlor., slow i.v. in 500 ml dextrose 5%". The ward stock cupboard contains only "dextrose 10%". Here the nurse is involved in both reducing the stock solution strength from 10% to 5% and also in using a height-weight nomogram to ascertain the body surface area, before calculating the dose. All the information is relevant at some stage. Particular care is needed with some modern drugs, especially cytotoxic and paediatric ones, for which the therapeutic level is close to the toxic dose.

These examples serve, too, to show the kinds of ratio and proportion problems which are crucial in all drug calculations.

5. Mastery

Nursing is a profession where decisions and calculations can be vital ones. Mention has been made of the upper bounds of difficulty in the various topics, but it is necessary to emphasise that in most areas, these bounds are also the desirable levels of mastery which a learner should achieve, to ensure that she will be a safe and capable nurse. That drug calculations need to be highly accurate should be obvious. Not so evident is that a less than perfect knowledge of the S.I. units within the stated bounds may lead a learner to conclude that since there are 100 cm in 1 m, there are also 100 micrograms in 1 mg, resulting in a dose 10 times too great. When dealing with indices, a nurse, who does not realise that the change from $4{\cdot}5 \times 10^{12}$ to $3{\cdot}5 \times 10^{12}$ in the number of red blood cells per litre is a fall of 1,000,000,000,000 cells, not 1 cell, may fail to alert the doctor to a serious change in the patient's condition. A badly plotted graph such as Insert 3.4 may hide symptom trends and lead to mis-diagnosis of the patient's condition (Pirie, 1981).

The desirable mastery levels for each topic are indicated in Insert 3.1 (column 2) and where these differ from the upper bounds, reasons are given.

Chapter 4 describes the testing of nurses for mathematical competence based on this taxonomy.

6. Summary

Using observational techniques, informal interviews with staff and learners, analysis of over 2,000 examination questions and of the content of the four British 'maths for nurses' textbooks available at that time, a list of 24 mathematical skills which are necessary to a nurse was composed. From the results of a questionnaire put to 18 nurse tutors and from the study of the observation schedules, upper bounds of difficulty and desired levels of mastery were defined. These topics and mastery levels were then used as the basis of tests which are described in Chapter 4.

CHAPTER 4

The Achievement Test and Self-assessment Survey

The second phase of the project was to look at the problems learner nurses were having with the mathematics in the taxonomy presented in Insert 3.1.

1. Objectives

The objectives at this stage were:

(i) to show that remediation in some of the mathematical topics is needed by a large number of learners;
(ii) to rate the difficulty to the learners of the 24 topics;
(iii) to determine whether performance in nursing mathematics correlates with stage of training, entry qualifications or status as a student or pupil;
(iv) to determine the awareness of learners of their own mathematical limitations.

2. Achievement Test Construction

Based on this 'maths for nurses' taxonomy, a set of behavioural objectives was composed (Insert 3.1, column 4) and a criterion-referenced test was written, to ascertain in which topics and to what extent learners were experiencing problems. Appendix B contains the final version of this test. The test initially contained one question with two parts on each topic: the first testing the fundamental rules of, say, subtraction of decimals with a straightforward example such as $0{\cdot}35-0{\cdot}07$, the second testing the topic at the upper range of the objective, say, subtraction of decimals with unequal number of decimal places, $0{\cdot}035-0{\cdot}0125$. This initial version was piloted on three volunteer learners and two nurses to obtain an idea of the time needed to complete such a test and to gain their opinions on the test content. As a result of this trial, six of the questions were reduced to one part only, with no loss of assessment (questions K on division by decimals, M on converting decimals to fractions, N on percentage, S on indices, T on decimal place value, X on negative numbers) and four others were restructured (questions P on S.I. units, R on use of tables, U on recording in tables, V on plotting graphs). This second version of the test was field trialed on two study groups of 15 and 17 learners, all of whom completed the test within one hour. An item analysis as recommended by Gronlund (1968a) was performed. None of the items produced a negative index of discrimination, although several of the indices were zero. This was to be expected, however, since the test did not aim to measure achievement relative to other learners, but relative to the criteria set by the mastery levels. All the learners completed (A) on addition of integers accurately, none had completely correct answers for the ratio and S.I. Units questions (O and P). The decision was taken, based on Gronlund (1968b), Popham and Husek (1969) and Popham (1978), not to exclude any of the items on the final version of the test. Since the content domain and item generation rules resulted from objectives, defined as recommended by Bormuth (1970), context validity could be assumed (Hambleton and Novick, 1973). Validity was further reinforced by comments on the test from two nurse tutors who were in agreement that the questions were appropriate and applicable to nurses.

The incorrect answers were analysed in detail to ascertain the types of errors being committed and this led to the wording in two of the questions being changed. "Drug" was substituted for "solute" in the ratio question (O), since it seemed possible that misunderstanding of the language may have led to some of the respondents giving the quantity of water needed. "You want" was used in preference for "requirement" in the formula questions (Q) since the skill being tested was simply one of substitution.

The test was intended to be used on between 500 and 600 learner nurses, and it was thus essential that marking should be as simple as possible. It was also the intention that the test be of a diagnostic nature to aid future remediation programmes. To these aims, Gronlund (1976) recommends the format of multiple choice. The distractors were chosen from the analysed erroneous answers of the trial group to ensure that they were appropriate to the level of ability of the future candidates. The danger of closed questions (Oppenheim, 1966) was guarded against by having a blank alternative box for each question and by using an early simple question (that is Question B(i) 75 − 56) to demonstrate the need to use the box for some questions (Marshall and Hales, 1971).

The disadvantage of criterion-referenced mastery tests is the difficulty of assessing the reliability of the instrument. No really satisfactory statistical solution has yet been achieved (Hambleton and Novick, 1973).

In this particular case, it was not instructive to look at internal consistency since the test was not intended to be in any way homogeneous.

Gronlund (1976) suggested that for very specific and highly structured outcomes five test items:

"may be sufficient for dependable judgement concerning mastery . . . however, ten items for each specific learning outcome would provide a more desirable minimum."

It was clearly impractical, in a test with the breadth of cover needed in this work, to follow this advice.

Ebel (1969) puts forward a formula for calculating the increase in reliability one can expect with an increase of choices per item. This is, however, based on the Kuder-Richardson formula 21 which assumes homogeneity in the test. It is reasonable to assume, nevertheless, that some increase in reliability is to be had by increasing the multiple choice distractors. Since it was possible to produce from the field trials at least four erroneous answers per part of each question, it was reasonable to offer six choices in most questions.

3. Self-assessment Survey Instrument

To attain objectives (iii) and (iv) given at the beginning of this Chapter, an instrument consisting of two components was designed. A short Biographic Inventory was followed by a section in which learners made a self-assessment of their ability to perform certain mathematical tasks. The final form of the instrument is given in Appendix C. The items in the self-assessment section were based on the 'maths-for-nurses' taxonomy in Insert 3.1. Learners were asked to rate, on a scale of 1–4, their ability to reach the required mastery level for each of the 24 topics. The definition of each category of the scale was very precisely explained as follows:

1. Easy means: could do it in my head; might need a scrap of paper; sure of how to do it; confident the answer will be right.
2. Fairly easy means: could probably do it given time; would definitely need paper or tables; reasonably sure I know how to do it; fairly confident the answer would be right.
3. Difficult means: would need some help; would need a calculator; not quite sure how to do it; would need to check with someone.
4. Impossible means: could not do it; would get someone to do it for me; have never understood this; don't know how to begin.

This survey was piloted and field-trialled in the same way as the Achievement Test. Validity was again assured by reference to the objectives. To assess the reliability of the survey 22 learners judged their abilities on two occasions, 10 days apart. Random ordering and re-ordering of the topics on the two survey forms was rejected as confusing and two different types of logical groupings were used instead. In the first survey the topics were grouped according to the types of numbers involved (integers, fractions, decimals etc.), in the second, they were grouped by operation (addition, subtraction, etc.). Of the 528 pairs (t_i, r_i) of test/retest scores, only 81 had $|t_i - r_i| > 0$, thus 85% of the assessments remained unchanged on the retest.[1]

4. Sample Selection and Test Administration

Although all students sit the same examination to qualify as State Registered Nurses, there is considerable difference between the Schools of Nursing on a variety of counts. Entry requirements range upwards from "3 O-level passes" to "2 A-levels preferred". Recruitment ranges from local to international. The setting for clinical experience ranges from small country hospitals to large prestigious teaching hospitals. The situation for pupils is similarly varied. To cover a broad spectrum of learners, four schools were chosen:

(i) a small school, requiring the minimum entry qualifications and recruiting mainly from the local area;
(ii) a medium-sized school requiring more than minimum entry standard and recruiting approximately 60% of its learners locally;
(iii) a large school requiring high entry standards and recruiting approximately 40% locally;
(iv) a large, prestigious school, training for specialist paediatric nursing stipulating mathematics O level at grade A, B or C, among its high entry requirements, and recruiting internationally.

From these hospitals, 22 groups of students and pupils, covering all stages of training, and containing 571 learners in total, were examined.

The examination lasted one and a half hours and was in two sections: the Self-assessment Survey Instrument, followed by the Achievement Test. Learners were unaware, when assessing their skills, that they would then be required to do a mathematical test, but it was stressed that the objective of the survey was to look for weaknesses in order to facilitate the provision of suitable remediation. It was hoped that this presentation would discourage them from underestimating (to cover themselves against a low mark in the Test) or over-estimating (to impress an outside researcher). Total confidentiality was assured.

5. Designing the Mark Scheme

Since the aim at this stage of the project was to be able to make certain predictions about learners based on the Achievement Test and

[1] The reliability of the instrument is demonstrated further by a related t-test on topic scores producing a value of $t = 1{\cdot}669$ which is not significant at the $0{\cdot}1$ level.

Self-assessment Survey, it was essential to devise a mark scheme for the test which related very closely to the 1–4 categories in the Self-assessment Survey.

Two types of error were first defined:

A fundamental error (F) is an error in the basic technique of the mathematical skill being tested by that particular question, e.g. Topic G, decimal addition $0{\cdot}24+0{\cdot}19=0{\cdot}33$. This demonstrates failure to 'carry' when calculating $4+9$.

A slip (sl) is an error which is non-fundamental to the skill being tested by a particular question, e.g. Topic X, negative numbers, $0{\cdot}24+0{\cdot}19+(-0{\cdot}2)=0{\cdot}13$. This comes from $0{\cdot}33-0{\cdot}2$ which is an error of decimal addition and not of negative number manipulation.

This led to the following basic rationale for scoring the test:

Score 1 if
- whole question correct ('sure of how to do it')
  - with no written working ('do it in my head')
  - with trivial written working ('might need a scrap of paper').

Score 2 if
- whole question correct, but
  - with heavy working ('definitely need paper')
  - with erroneous attempts ('probably do it given time')
- or there is a slip in one part ('fairly confident').

Score 3 if
- part of the question correct, but
  - one part fundamentally wrong ('not quite sure how to do it')
  - one part omitted ('need some help/calculator')
- or there is a slip in both parts ('need someone to check it').

Score 4 if
- whole question wrong ('could not do it')
- or omitted ('get someone else to do it'/'don't know how to begin').

Five of the questions P, R, U, V, W were deemed to need marking on a proportional basis. Two mathematicians having discussed the marking rationale and the definition of slip versus fundamental error, independently drew up a mark scheme for each of the 24 test questions. These schemes were in 93% agreement, the differences being over what constituted 'heavy working' in questions A and B, what category of answer '031' in question D fell into, and whether a wrong operation, for example, add instead of subtract, was a slip or a fundamental error. After further discussion, these differences were resolved; '031' was categorised as "correct with heavy working". Since the learners themselves were numbered 01, 02, etc. on the test paper, it was felt that one could not call 031 incorrect even though it did display a probable lack of understanding of the answer. Wrong operations were counted as fundamental errors, even if the correct operation was used elsewhere, in questions where it was obvious from the magnitude or nature of the answer that it must be incorrect, for example, $75-56 = 131$. The estimation of a 'likely' answer should be a part of every nurse's armour against errors. It was not possible to detect from this test how many learners did assess their answers for 'reasonableness', but it is suspected that in fact the number was very small.

Using the revised mark scheme, the two mathematicians independently marked 44 scripts and these were compared, question for question, to test the ability of the mark scheme to define, uniquely, a mark for any answers, or answer combination, for each question. Out of 1,066 answers, 23 discrepencies were found. Of these, 14 were due to errors by the markers and 9 due to different interpretations of unforeseen errors, 7 of them in question V. The mark scheme for V was expanded to include these errors. The mark scheme could thus be considered unambiguous on a minimum of 99·16% of the questions. This was considered sufficiently accurate for the scheme to be used to mark the whole sample tested. It was felt, too, that an examiner's marking error rate of 1·313% was tolerable.

6. Results

Insert 4.1 presents the rounded percentages of 1 to 4 scores for each topic on the mathematics Achievement Test.

It should be borne in mind when considering these results, that a score of 1 indicates mastery and a score of 4 represents total inability to answer the question correctly. Thus the higher the scores, the greater the need for remediation. The data, however, cannot be treated as other than ordinal. That remediation treatment is desirable for many of the learners in some topics is crudely indicated by the very low percentage achieving mastery (5% for P) and high percentage totally failing (51% for K and S) in some topics.

The trial marking of question V had indicated some unexpected errors and analysis of the whole sample showed that there were indeed many difficulties in allocating the scores to the solutions of this question and question W which depended upon it. One of the major problems was that misplotting in V eliminated some of the deliberate distractors in the answering of W, and a new mark scheme had to be devised to cope with this situation.

It was decided that although there was definite evidence of inability by some learners to read and plot graphs, questions V and W could not accurately be ranked with the other questions. These were, therefore, dropped from the investigation. The whole field of graphs in nursing needs further exploration.

Insert 4.1:
Achievement Score Distribution

Topic	Percentages of Scores 1	2	3	4		
A	71	25	4	0	+	Integers
B	45	41	13	1	−	
C	42	45	12	1	×	
D	48	15	35	2	÷	
E	47	19	20	14	+	Fractions
F	22	23	11	44	×	
G	67	25	8	1	+	Decimals
H	22	33	28	17	−	
I	19	46	29	6	×	
J	20	12	47	21	÷	
K	23	18	8	51	÷	
L	25	10	30	35	Decimals ⟷ Fractions	
M	55	5	11	29		
N	53	14	2	31	%	
O	12	3	44	41	Ratio	
P	5	22	37	36	S.I. Units	
Q	43	6	16	35	Formulae	
R	58	30	4	7	Printed tables	
S	35	3	11	51	Indices	
T	80	2	8	10	Place value	
U	91	2	1	6	Tabular recording	
V	34	18	19	29	Plot	Graphs
W	18	4	13	65	Interpret	
X	25	11	22	42	Negative numbers	

7. Areas of Difficulty

Three separate methods were used to rank the topics in order of difficulty to the learners:

(i) 'Lack of mastery' shown by the percentage of learners failing to achieve a 1-score.
(ii) 'Complete failure' shown by the percentage of learners obtaining a 4-score.
(iii) 'Experiencing difficulty' shown by the percentage of learners obtaining a 3- or a 4-score.

Insert 4.2 gives the rank order of the topics using these three methods.

From consideration of the first ten items in the Insert, seven topics—F, K, L, O, P, S, X: fraction multiplication, decimal division by decimal, fraction/decimal conversion, ratio, S.I. Units, indices,

Insert 4.2:
Topics Ranked for Difficulty

Rank	Lack of Mastery	%	Complete failure	%	Experiencing difficulty	%
1	P	95	K, S	51	O	85
2	O	88	—		P	73
3	I	81	F	44	J	68
4	J	80	X	42	L	65
5	F, H	78	O	41	X	64
6	—		P	36	S	62
7	K	77	L, Q	35	K	59
8	L, X	75	—		F	55
9	—		N	31	Q	51
10	S	65	M	29	H	45
11	C	58	J	21	M	40
12	Q	57	H	17	D	37
13	B	55	E	14	I	35
14	E	53	T	10	E	34
15	D	52	R	7	N	33
16	N	47	I, U	6	T	18
17	M	45	—		B	14
18	R	42	D	2	C	13
19	G	33	G, B, C	1	R	11
20	A	29	—		G	9
21	T	20	—		U	7
22	U	9	A	0	A	4

Insert 4.3: Test Grades Related to GCE and CSE Qualifications

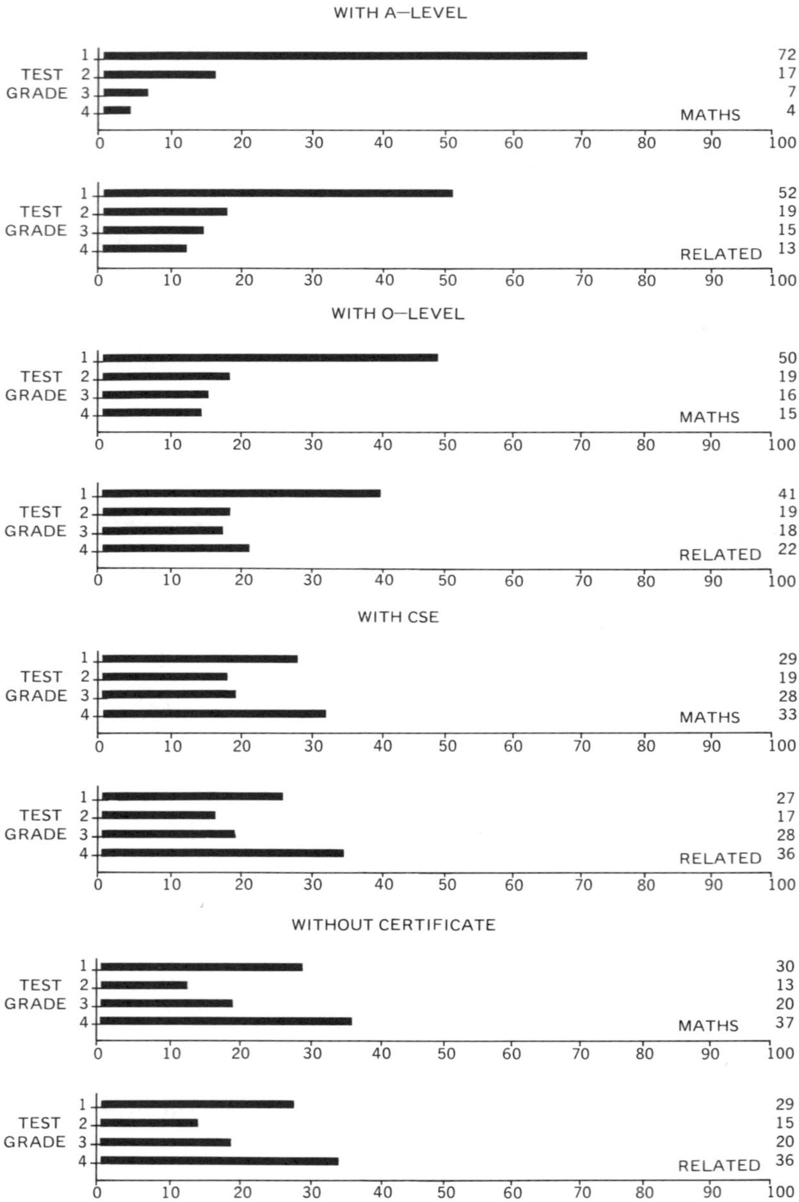

negative numbers—are clearly indicated by all three ranking methods as having been poorly done in the Achievement Test. In fact, with the exception of addition of decimals (G), all the decimal arithmetic questions (H to M) occur at least once in the top ten of the difficulty ratings. More than half of the tested sample had problems with formulae (Q) and nearly one third completely failed the question on percentages (N).

One area, more than any other, where accuracy is vital is in the calculation and administration of drug doses. The mathematical skills involved in this task are those of ratio (O), S.I. Units (P), division of integers and decimals (D, J, K), selection of data and use of formulae (Q), occasionally percentages (N) and, for checking calculations an idea of the 'size' of a decimal (T). Of these topics only D and T do not appear in the top ten of any of the rank orders. This was thus clearly a nursing area which, both in terms of importance and of mathematical skill deficiency, merited remedial attention.

At the other end of the scale, learners seem to be reasonably competent in integer arithmetic (A, B, C, D), use of printed tables (R) and recording information in tabular form (U). It is arguable that the facility with which learners handle conversion tables is itself a reason for their lack of knowledge of the International Units System. Further specific investigations would be needed, however, to confirm this theory.

8. Performance Correlation with Year of Training

The scores for the topics are taken over a complete range of year groups, so one must consider whether learners in fact 'pick-up as they go along' the skills they need. The frequencies of "1" scores for students and pupils across the year groups were examined separately. Details of the statistical tests used are given in Insert 4.8 and the related text at the end of this Chapter.[2]

The results showed that one cannot rely on learners to absorb the required mathematics "by osmosis" from their surroundings.

9. Performance Correlations with GCE and CSE Grades

Since ability in nursing mathematics does not correlate significantly with year of study it seems prudent to investigate whether it is possible to predict which learners will have problems.

Insert 4.3 shows the percentage of learners averaged over the 22

[2] The frequencies of '1' scores for 452 Students across the year groups are given in Insert 4.8. The data categories are discrete and the three year-samples independent, therefore the chi-squared test for significant differences can be applied to test the null hypothesis that frequency of 1-scores is not related to the number of years spent in training. The expected frequencies are marked thus *.

topics, who attained each score. The learners are partitioned by qualification (A-level, O-level, CSE, without certificate), firstly in mathematics and secondly in the mathematics related subjects of physics, chemistry, economics, geography and engineering. OND was considered equivalent to A level.

From this visual presentation, it can readily be seen that those learners with A-level mathematics achieve considerably more '1' scores than any other group, with only 11% experiencing difficulty in any topic. A-level 'related subjects' and O-level mathematics produce very similar score distributions, with approximately one third of the students having difficulties in some area. The distribution pattern for both the CSE and the 'without certificate' groups appear very similar. In these groups, over half the learners have experienced difficulties, and one third have completely failed in some nursing mathematics topic.

Although one can predict that students with A-level mathematics will find little difficulty with the mathematics needed for nursing, all other learners will need a substantial degree of remedial teaching. ***Thus entry qualifications other than A-level mathematics do not provide a particularly useful prediction of the need for remediation.***

10. Performance Correlation with Status—Student or Pupil

Insert 4.4 shows the percentage of learners attaining each grade, partitioned by status—Student or Pupil.

It can be seen from comparison of the percentages of learners achieving '1' scores (45% students, 27% pupils) and also of those with '4' scores (18% students, 37% pupils) that, as a group, the students are better at nursing mathematics than the pupils. This was to be expected. Nevertheless, it is also evident that a large percentage of the students do need some remedial help.

Insert 4.4: Test Grades Related to Status

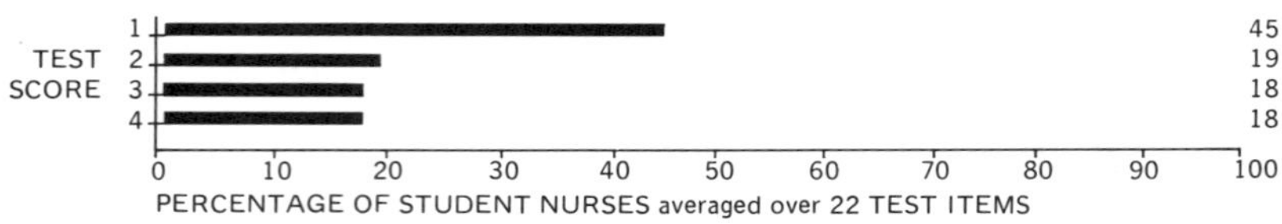

TEST SCORES of PUPIL NURSES

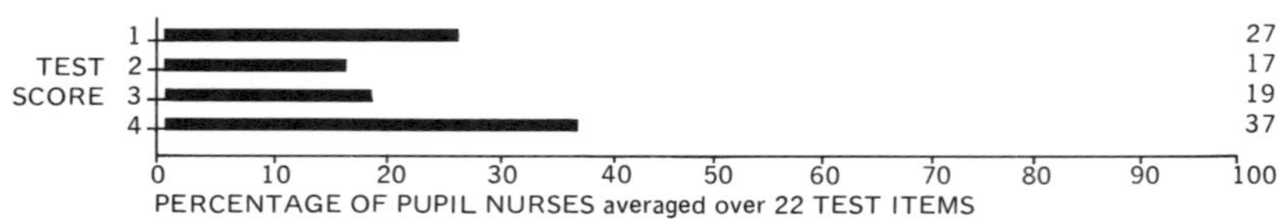

Insert 4.5:
Self-assessed Score Distribution

Topic	Percentages of Scores			
	1	2	3	4
A	98	2	0	0
B	94	6	0	0
C	77	22	0	0
D	56	41	3	0
E	50	37	11	2
F	37	43	18	2
G	78	18	3	0
H	65	28	6	1
I	39	48	12	2
J	28	49	20	3
K	23	43	28	5
L	23	41	29	8
M	42	40	14	4
N	50	39	11	0
O	24	43	27	6
P	16	40	31	13
Q	22	51	22	5
R	57	32	9	3
S	40	28	22	10
T	75	17	6	2
U	76	21	3	0
V	86	13	1	0
W	87	12	1	0
X	41	40	16	3

Insert 4.6: Comparison of Self-Assessment and Achievement Test Scores

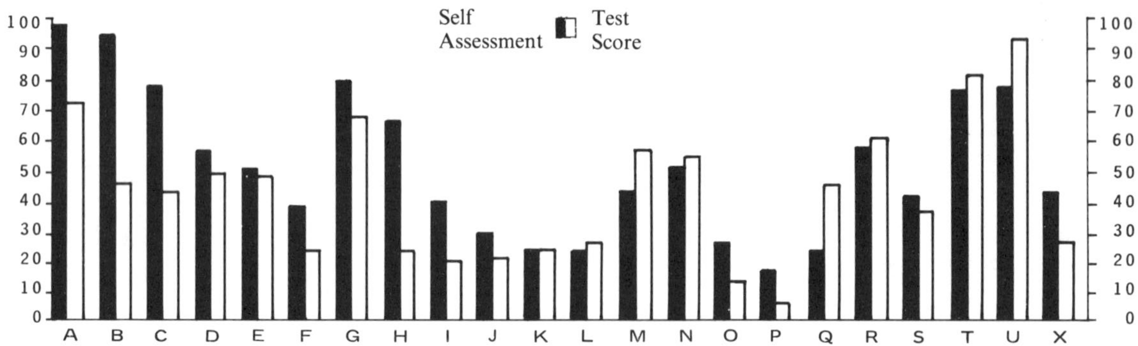

1 — SCORES

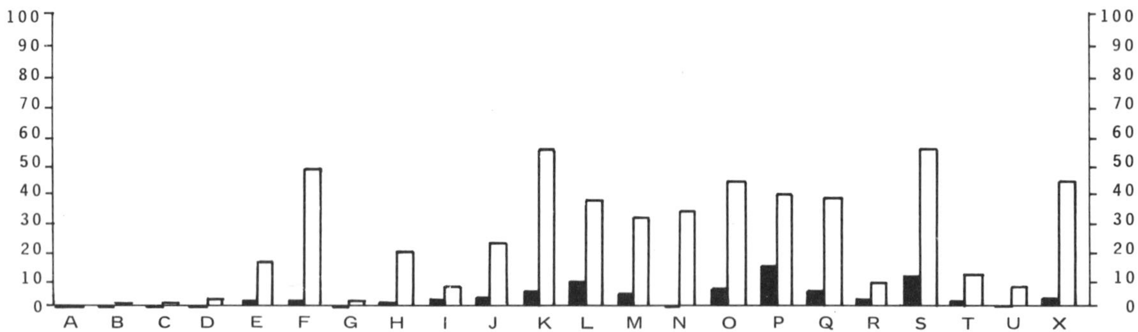

4 — SCORES

11. Self-assessment

The simplest method of allocating remediation would be by self-selection. This is only a viable proposition, however, if learners are aware of their problems. Insert 4.5 presents the Self-assessed Score distribution in the same format as Insert 4.1 (Achievement Score distribution). The tables are by no means identical. This can be seen more clearly in Insert 4.6, where the actual and assessed scores (excluding topics V and W for the reasons given earlier in the Chapter) have been plotted for '1' scores and for '4' scores.

It is evident that for '1' scores, not only do the 'assessed' and 'achieved' not coincide, but the learners also do not consistently over- or under-estimate their abilities. The '4' score profile, however reveals substantial underestimation of the difficulty of almost all topics. To examine the relationship between the actual and assessed score for each individual on each topic, a 4 × 4 grid was drawn up and each score pair—achieved against assessed—was plotted. Insert 4.7 summarises the grid, by giving the rounded percentage in each cell. The shaded cells highlight the accurate assessments.

The variation in ability to assess their skills is not peculiar to nurses, but accords with the findings of a range of literature reviewed in Chapter 2.

Since overestimation of abilities by almost one half of the learners would probably lead to them not seeking the mathematical help they need, ***self-selection cannot be considered a satisfactory basis on which to allocate remediation.***

The final section of the research investigated the use of a diagnostic test and various remedial teaching methods. The methodology and results are set out in Chapters, 5, 6 and 7.

Insert 4.7:
Comparison of Achieved and Assessed Scores

		Achieved 1	2	3	4
Assessed	1	28	11	7	8
	2	10	6	8	8
	3	2	1	2	6
	4	0	0	1	2

Summary of Ability Estimations

48% overestimate
38% are accurate
14% underestimate

Insert 4.8:
Distribution of '1' Scores by Year Group

			YEAR GROUP 1	2	3	Total
Score Frequency	1-score	Actual	2527	1258	972	4757
		Expected	2547*	1284*	926*	
	Not 1-score	Actual	3281	1670	1140	6091
		Expected	3261*	1644*	1186*	
		Total	5808	2928	2112	10848

$\chi^2 = 5{\cdot}2866$ and is not significant at 0·05 level, so that *one cannot rely on the Student learning the required mathematics 'by osmosis'. A similar finding pertains to Pupils.*

12. Summary

This extensive Chapter has described the construction of an Achievement Test, based on the taxonomy in Chapter 3, its implementation, and its marking. A Self-assessment Survey was also devised to investigate the awareness of learners of their own mathematical weaknesses. Four Schools of Nursing were selected for testing and 571 learners across all three years of training took part in the project. The results are presented and ways of rating the topics for difficulty are discussed. *A conclusion that there are certain specified topics in which many learners need remedial teaching is drawn.*

Consideration of the mastery scores across the three years of training indicates that *learners cannot be relied on to "pick up" the mathematical skill which they need as they go along.* In addition, although there exists some correlation between external qualifications in mathematics and performance in the Achievement Test, *the qualifications cannot be considered particularly useful predictors of the need for remediation. Learners are also shown to be inconsistent and inaccurate in their assessment of their own skills and, therefore, self-selection would not be an ideal method of allocating mathematical help.*

CHAPTER 5

Designing the Teaching Materials and Diagnostic Test

The previous Chapter has indicated that it is desirable for most learners to be given some help with the mathematics needed for their careers. Stage 3 of the investigation was, therefore, to consider various possible remedial instruction methods. This Chapter discusses the preparation of the necessary materials and diagnostic test.

1. Topic Selection

Five groups of topics from the mathematics taxonomy (Chapter 3) were selected with reference to the results of the Achievement Test (Chapter 4) to form the basis of an experiment to compare remedial methods. These were:

(i) Ratio (O) and decimal division (K) and (J)—all crucial to drug dosage calculations.
(ii) S.I. Units (P)—essential for all nursing measurements.
(iii) Formulae (Q)—used in drug and dietary calculations, and frequently in paediatric work.
(iv) Percentages (N)—and limited conversion of fractions to decimals (L) occurring in drug and solution calculations, and in ward and laboratory diagnostic testing.
(v) Indices (S)—necessary for the interpretation of laboratory reports.

Negative numbers (X) and fractions (F) and (M), although ranking high in the difficulty rating, were considered less vital skills and, therefore, not singled out for treatment on this occasion.

2. Objectives

The literature reviewed in Chapter 2 indicated that self-instructional materials can form a powerful teaching tool. Before this method could be monitored within the experiment, however, some suitable texts had to be written. Thus the first objective of Stage 3 was to produce and pilot five self-help, nursing orientated booklets on drug doses, S.I. Units, formulae, percentages and indices. The second objective was to produce and pilot a Diagnostic Test to enable learners to decide in which mathematical areas they needed help.

3. Writing the Booklets

There are five main stages in the composition of instructional materials:

1. Define the behavioural objectives.
2. Decide on methodology and presentation.
3. Analyse and organise the subject matter.
4. Draft and pilot the materials.
5. Validate the final product.

The objectives for each booklet were based on the upper bounds of the relevant topics and stated in each introduction. The intention was to keep the material as closely related as possible to the nursing context.

Each of the topics lent itself readily to division into simple sequential stages. The style of presentation chosen, however, was not that of 'single frame' programmed learning, but was based on Gilbert's advocation (1978) that as many stimuli as the student can cope with should be grouped together. Thus the text takes the learner systematically through a situation with examples worked in detail before posing some similar questions to be answered. The associated arithmetic necessary for calculation, but not crucial to understanding the method, is treated in the text in the form of revisional material and inserted when needed. The decision on what arithmetic needed revising was taken independently in each booklet and based on the product theorem "performance need for that topic x student deficiency = coverage" (Gilbert, 1978). The student deficiency was based on the results of the Achievement Test.

Two major check-tests are included, one part-way through the booklet (Re-cap Check) and one at the end (Final Check) and references are given with the answers to enable learners to trace the section of the text relevant to any errors they may have made.

Formative evaluation of the materials was provided by a group of qualified nurses and a separate group of first-year learners, who read and discussed the texts, and by four nurse tutors who individually provided comments. Various changes, such as the deletion of reference to a drug no longer available, were made as a result.

The final versions of the booklets used in the remediation experiment have now been published by Baillière Tindall as a book entitled "Maths for Nursing". An extract from one of the booklets is given in Appendix D.

4. Composing and Validating the Diagnostic Test

A Diagnostic Test was then designed to cover the topics selected for inclusion in the remediation experiment. The intention was to produce a multidimensional test made up of unidimensional sub-tests, each sub-test related to the criteria for topic mastery levels given in the taxonomy in Chapter 3. Cronbach and Glaser (1965) recommended that the testing time be split equally between topics, if future decisions are to be made by giving equal weight to each subtest. Since in this case the decisions for remediation would be made independently for each sub-test, it was considered more appropriate to hold the number of questions constant, rather than the time allowed:

> "The problem of how to fix the length of each subscale so as to maximise the percentage of correct decisions . . . on the basis of the test results has yet to be resolved," (Hambleton and Novick, 1973).

and so the decision of six items per topic was made based on the assumption that learners could complete the total test within one hour. An hour was selected as the optimum total test length, as longer might discourage tutors from incorporating the test in the crowded introductory block timetable, and less time would restrict the diagnostic range of the questions. Each of the five sections, therefore, contained six questions, ordered so that a learner would be able to identify the topics, or areas within a topic, where mistakes were occurring. Multiple choice was not considered an appropriate format, because the diagnostic element was built into the sequence of six questions rather than into a variety of responses to one question.

Twenty-eight learners were tested using the 'experiment version' of the test, and retested using the same test eight days later. On both occasions all the learners completed the test well within the hour. The reliability of this test was shown by a correlation coefficient of 0·9443 which is significant at the 0·001 level. An item analysis revealed one question (on formulae) with negative discrimination, and one (on indices) with zero discrimination.

The first formula question was

$$\text{"Given: mean} = \frac{\text{sum of values}}{\text{number of values}}$$

find the mean, if 5 values have a sum of 100".

Discussion with the learners produced the information that many of them had not regarded the question as a case of simple substitution, but had reacted to the word 'mean' with feelings such as "I can't do statistics", and had, therefore, not attempted a solution. Further evidence of this phenomenon is discussed in Pirie (1981). This question was subsequently replaced by one on petrol consumption.

Scrutiny of the answers to the dubious index question showed that learners were able to rank order 4^3, 2^3, 1^3 correctly, while still believing $2^3 = 6$ and $1^3 = 3$. The '1^3' was replaced by '1^9' in the final version of the test. The problem of selecting appropriate mastery scores has been discussed in Chapter 2. The restriction of only six questions per topic, however, inhibited the adoption of a 90% correct score. With reference to the taxonomy in Chapter 3, therefore, five out of six correct responses were deemed a mastery score, in the formulae and indices sub-tests, where the mastery level needed was lower than the upper bound (see Chapter 3), while six correct responses were required to achieve mastery scores for drug doses, S.I. Units and percentages.

The revised booklets and the Diagnostic Test then formed part of the experiment designed to investigate various instructional methods and described in the following Chapter.

5. Summary

Five areas of nursing mathematics, (drug doses, S.I. units, indices, formulae and percentages) were identified as needing remedial teaching to large numbers of learners, and selected to form the basis of an experiment to examine various remediation methods. Self-instructional booklets were written and piloted on these topics. A Diagnostic Test, based on a universe-defined test was constructed, validated, piloted and verified for reliability, to assess learning in the above topics.

Since the test was being designed not only for use on one research occasion, but was intended to be an integral part of any remediation programme, incorporating successive re-testing where expedient, it was necessary to formulate some method of replicability of test items. Osburn (1968) proposed a 'universe-defined' Achievement Test which is:

> "constructed and administered in such a way that the examinee's score on the test provides an unbiased estimate of his score on some explicitly defined universe of item content."

Content validity, generalisability and consistency are thus ensured, provided the items in a particular test are selected by stratified random sampling from the universe of content. To fulfil these conditions a technique similar to that reported by Hively *et al.* (1968) was used and diagnostic categories were delineated and generalised items constructed. From these item specifications, an actual test was produced for use in the experiment. A sample of these items, together with the final version of the test used, are given in Appendix E.

CHAPTER 6

The Experiment to Compare Various Methods of Remediation

The aim of the third stage of the work was to compare the efficacy of several different forms of mathematical remediation available to nurses. This Chapter describes these methods of remediation and provides the rationale underlying the experiment designed to test their power to effect improvement in nursing learners' mathematical skills.

1. Remediation Options

Remediation could be at one of three levels:

(a) Class teaching when the learners are in block.
(b) Individual tuition by: (i) a tutor; (ii) specially designed self-instructional materials; (iii) externally motivated use of text-books and media.
(c) Assimilation during practical work on the course, together with self-motivated use of available resources.

It proved impossible to evaluate the potential for improvement due to class teaching, since none of the Schools of Nursing approached were willing to organise the necessary time in an already tightly structured learners' time-table. Indeed, although genuine concern over learners' failings exists, on the whole, as Dexter and Applegate (1980) wrote:

> "the nursing faculty does not view its role as tutors in basic maths."

This in no way diminishes the value of the research, since it indicates that class teaching is not, in practical terms, a viable remedial option. Similarly individual tuition by a tutor was not a feasible proposition.

It was not possible to test learning of type (c) unaffected by the influence of a pre-test, since without a pre-test the experimental groups could not be judged for homogeneity. It had already been established in Stage 2 (Chapter 4) however, that learners, who had not been alerted to their mathematical difficulties, could not be relied upon to pick up the necessary mathematical skills as they went along.

2. The Experimental Design

The final objective of the research was thus to construct, conduct, and analyse the results of an experiment to compare the effects of remediation at levels b (ii), (self-instructional materials), b (iii) (externally motivated use of test books) and c (natural assimilation plus pre-test).

Two learner groups were given certain treatments, and a third group acted as a control group.

The experimental design used is best explained diagramatically in Insert 6.1.

Insert 6.1:
Experimental Design on Effects of Remediation

Group	Day 1	Day 2			Treatment Days 2–26			Day 27	Day 28
H_1	P_r	F_{Pr}	B_{T1} + time	B_{T2}	—	L_{T4}	B_{T5}	P_o	F_{Po}
H_2	P_r	F_{Pr}	B_{T1}	L_{T2}	B_{T3}	B_{T4}	—	P_o	F_{Po}
H_3	P_r	F_{Pr}	—	—	—	—	—	P_o	F_{Po}

where H_i is a group of learners (i = 1 to 3)
P_r is the pre-test
P_o is the post-test
F is the feedback
B is a self-instructional booklet (remediation level b (ii))
T_i is a nursing mathematics topic (i = 1 to 5)
L is a reading list (remediation level b (iii))
— is no treatment (remediation level c)
'time' is special study time allocated

3. Sample Selection

It was not practicable to assign learners randomly from one hospital group to the three experimental groups, since there was no way of preventing contamination between the treatments. Three Schools of Nursing were, therefore, selected to be as homogeneous as possible, on the basis of the same entry requirements—four O-levels for students, two for pupils; similar size—350 to 400 learners; similar recruiting ratios—40% local, 60% national; and similar local social environment. Learners in the introductory block were used for the experiment in order to avoid the effects of any teaching or ward experience not common to all the learners.

4. Testing and Feedback

The Diagnostic Test described in Chapter 5 was used for both pre-test and post-test. The pre-test was presented as normal procedure for new entrants, and learners were informed that they would be tested again four weeks later. Experimental mortality was nil.

After the pre-test, the test papers were returned to the learners who were encouraged to look at their scores and errors. Emphasis was laid on the need in nursing for accuracy and examples of medical uses for each of the topics were given. The test papers were then collected back and the appropriate booklets and printed reading lists given out.

Feedback is an essential component of a learning situation and, therefore, although unnecessary from the point of view of the experiment, feedback was also given on the post-test, in the form of detailed discussion between examiner and learners of the test questions, remedial methods and topics. Some of the learners' comments at this session are considered in Chapter 8.

5. Treatments

TOPICS

The five selected topics, referred to as T_i were

Drug doses	—T_1
S.I. units	—T_2
Formulae	—T_3
Percentages	—T_4
Indices	—T_5

BOOKLETS: B_{T1}–B_{T5} (level b (ii))

The booklets discussed in Chapter 5 were used to investigate the effect of self-instructional materials.

READING LIST: L_{T2} and L_{T4} (level b (iii))

A list of appropriate references in British mathematics-for-nursing textbooks was compiled, bearing in mind Hogstel's comment (1976) that a:

> "few essential references are much more effective than a long bibliography which often decreases a student's incentive."

There were no suitable television or radio programmes available at the time of testing.

NO TREATMENT: (level c + pre-test)

This was the status quo in all three schools; no teaching on any of the topics was time-tabled. Since tutors can be considered as valuable 'resources', they agreed to answer any questions concerning those topics not being treated with a booklet or reading list. Learners seeking help with the treated topics, however, would merely be referred back to the appropriate booklet or reading list.

6. Rationale of the Design

The control group H_3 was introduced to enable account to be taken of any learning occurring either naturally during the introductory block, or as a result of the pre-test. It was expected that the results would show that merely making learners aware of their deficiencies would be insufficient to engender significant learning.

Both group H_1 and H_2 were given the same booklet on Drug Doses (T_1), and had similar overall study time. Arrangements were made, however, for group H_1 to have a supervised period allotted specifically for the study of this booklet, in order to test the findings of Loughlin *et al.* (1964) who observed that supervised study periods did not improve study patterns or produce higher achievement levels.

The effects of using reading lists L_{T2} and L_{T4} for S.I. units (T_2) and percentages (T_4) were tested against the effects of providing the appropriate booklets B_{T2} and B_{T4}. The between-groups cross-over design for T_2 and T_4 was introduced to elicit any undesired effects of within-school attitude to, or accessibility of, the nursing library. It was thought that learners would learn less when expected to follow up suggested reading, than when given specific texts.

A similar design was used to test the remediation impact, in the cases of T_3 and T_5, of the booklets as compared with no treatment. It was considered possible that the environment of mathematical learning for groups H_1 and H_2 might cause some incidental transfer to the untreated topics.

The prime intention was to investigate the numbers of nurses reaching the specified mastery levels (Chapter 5) in the various topics, but by also considering all the score changes, information could be obtained about the general effects of the treatments. The results and their analyses are discussed in the next chapter.

7. Summary

An experiment was designed to test the relative effectiveness of three forms of remediation:

1. specially designed self-help materials
2. a short, relevant reading list
3. no treatment except the effects of the pre-test.

The five questions which it was hoped to answer were:

1. Is it sufficient for significant learning to take place, merely to make learners aware of their weaknesses?
2. Is the use of self-help booklets a more effective learning method than a reading list?
3. Is a reading list better than no treatment?
4. Does mathematical teaching in some topics motivate students to learn in other specified topic areas?
5. Does supervised study increase learning?

CHAPTER 7

The Results of the Remediation Experiment

The Diagnostic Test described in Chapter 5 was used for both pre- and post-testing for all students. It consisted of six questions on each of five topics, T_1–T_5. In the analysis which follows, learners' scores ranging from 0 to 6 are considered for each topic independently, so that the different treatments can be examined. The experimental design and mastery level scores, explained in Chapters 5 and 6, are repeated here for reference.

Group	Treatment				
H_1	B_{T1} + time	B_{T2}	—	L_{T4}	B_{T5}
H_2	B_{T1}	L_{T2}	B_{T3}	B_{T4}	—
H_3	—	—	—	—	—

T_1—mastery score = 6
T_2—mastery score = 6
T_3—mastery score = 5
T_4—mastery score = 6
T_5—mastery score = 5

In this Chapter the test results are presented diagrammatically both as histograms showing the frequencies of scores for the pre- and post-test (Insert 7.1) and as scatter-plots highlighting the change in scores of individual learners (Insert 7.2). There is a discussion of the statistical tests to be used in the subsequent analysis and the homogeneity of the three groups is demonstrated. The questions posed in the summary of Chapter 6 are then considered and following the analysis of the results, the conclusions reached are presented in bold type. Readers interested in the results rather than the statistical methods are invited to skim this Chapter noting those passages in bold type.

1. The Diagnostic Test Score Frequencies

Insert 7.1 shows the spread of scores for each group for the pre- and post-tests in each topic. For ease of visual comparison the post-test scores for topics treated with the booklets are contained in black boxes.

Insert 7.1: Diagnostic Test Results

TOPIC T1

	SCORE	PRE- NUMBER OF OBSERVATIONS	POST- NUMBER OF OBSERVATIONS
H1	0	0	0
	1	0	0
	2	6	2
	3	16	4
	4	13	7
	5	10	15
	6	3	20
H2	0	0	0
	1	2	2
	2	7	3
	3	10	6
	4	12	8
	5	16	20
	6	5	13
H3	0	0	0
	1	2	2
	2	8	7
	3	9	8
	4	14	18
	5	14	9
	6	3	6

TOPIC T2

	SCORE	PRE- NUMBER OF OBSERVATIONS	POST- NUMBER OF OBSERVATIONS
H1	0	32	6
	1	8	3
	2	6	6
	3	1	6
	4	1	5
	5	0	13
	6	0	8
H2	0	37	18
	1	10	12
	2	3	7
	3	1	6
	4	1	3
	5	0	4
	6	0	2
H3	0	36	27
	1	8	10
	2	3	9
	3	2	2
	4	0	1
	5	0	1
	6	1	1

TOPIC T3

	SCORE	PRE- NUMBER OF OBSERVATIONS	POST- NUMBER OF OBSERVATIONS
H1	0	1	1
	1	3	4
	2	6	4
	3	18	17
	4	11	6
	5	7	10
	6	2	6
H2	0	0	0
	1	7	2
	2	11	7
	3	5	8
	4	14	10
	5	11	11
	6	4	14
H3	0	0	0
	1	5	3
	2	11	12
	3	11	14
	4	11	12
	5	6	7
	6	5	3

TOPIC T4

	SCORE	PRE- NUMBER OF OBSERVATIONS	POST- NUMBER OF OBSERVATIONS
H1	0	3	2
	1	10	6
	2	10	6
	3	10	9
	4	10	13
	5	2	7
	6	3	5
H2	0	3	0
	1	15	2
	2	8	6
	3	14	9
	4	6	13
	5	3	10
	6	3	12
H3	0	2	6
	1	12	11
	2	12	11
	3	10	7
	4	8	9
	5	3	5
	6	3	2

TOPIC T5

	SCORE	PRE- NUMBER OF OBSERVATIONS	POST- NUMBER OF OBSERVATIONS
H1	0	8	0
	1	8	1
	2	4	1
	3	7	3
	4	5	5
	5	8	9
	6	8	29
H2	0	9	8
	1	6	5
	2	8	7
	3	8	7
	4	7	12
	5	6	7
	6	8	6
H3	0	8	5
	1	8	2
	2	8	7
	3	8	11
	4	6	9
	5	2	9
	6	10	7

Insert 7.2 Individual Learners' Scores

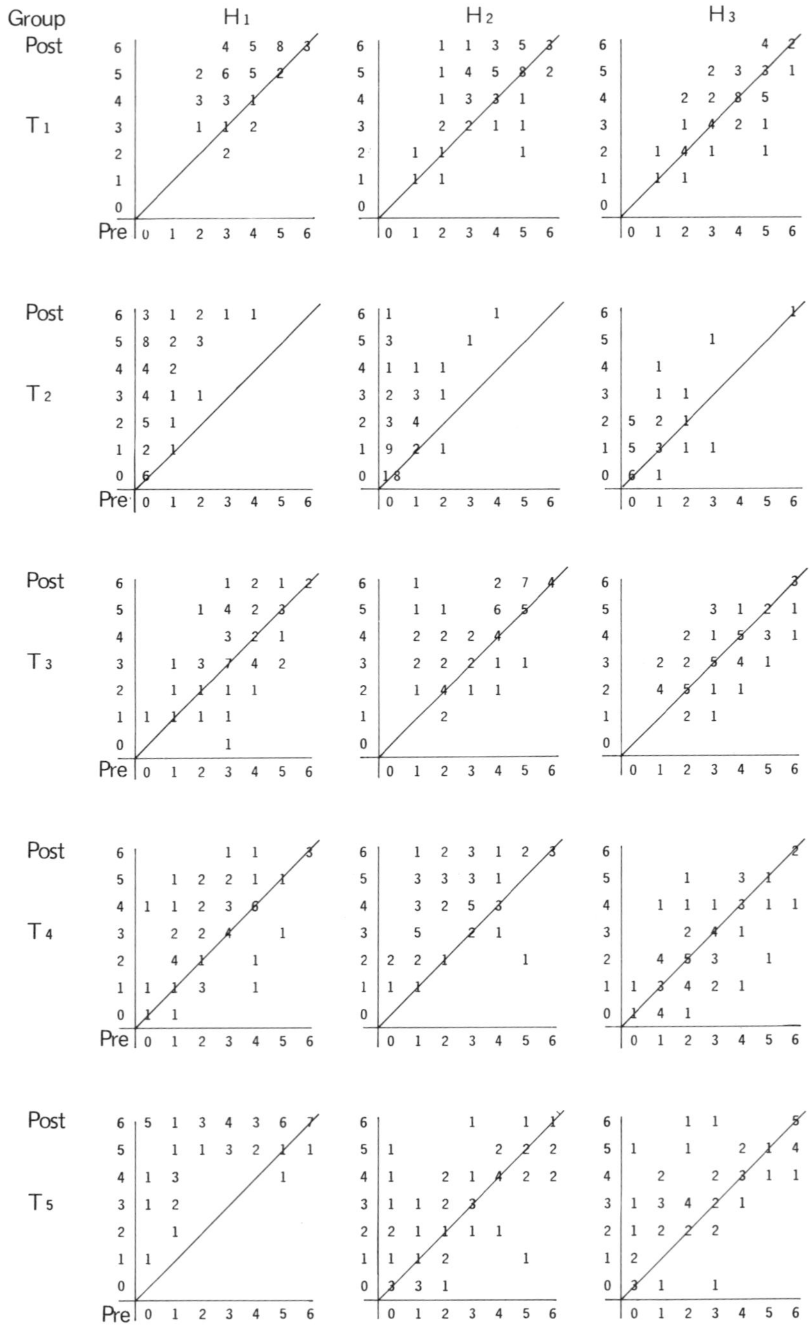

2. Selection of Appropriate Statistical Tests

From consideration of the pre-scores it is apparent that the scores for the sample selected are not normally distributed with respect to ability in the five tested topics. This is particularly noticeable in topics T_2 and T_5: T_2 being positively skewed, and T_5 showing a rectangular distribution, in all three groups. In the absence of any other research in this field, it was felt that one could not, therefore, assume that the sample had been selected from a population whose mathematical scores would be normally distributed. Thus one of the assumptions which underlies the use of parametric tests had not been met. In this situation, Siegel (1956) maintains that it is:

> "difficult to estimate the extent to which a probability statement is meaningful when (it) results from the unacceptable application of a (statistical) test."

An analysis, therefore, which does not make parametric assumptions is appropriate.

The actual scores fell into discrete categories measured on an ordinal scale, but an underlying continuum of mathematical ability was assumed to exist. The three groups were considered to be independent.

3. The Homogeneity of the Samples

The homogeneity of the three groups was investigated[(1)] and it was shown to be realistic to assume that the three sample groups were drawn from the same population and no allowances for pre-treatment differences need to be made. ***In the analysis which follows it is possible to make comparisons between the post-test scores for the three groups, knowing any differences which are observed cannot be considered due to pre-existing group differences.***

4. The Diagnostic Test Scores

Insert 7.2 displays individual learners' scores plotted pre-test against post-test. A number, say z, at the co-ordinate point (x, y) indicates

---

[(1)] To investigate the homogeneity of the three groups, the Kruskal-Wallis one-way analysis of variance by ranks was used on the pre-test scores with an allowance for tied scores, separately for each topic. This technique tests the null hypothesis that the samples come from the same population with respect to central tendency. The hypothesis for each of the topics T_1 to T_5 could not be rejected at the significance levels $\alpha = 0{\cdot}98, 0{\cdot}99, 0{\cdot}2, 0{\cdot}8, 0{\cdot}8$ respectively. Thus it was reasonable to assume that H_1, H_2, H_3 were drawn from the same population with respect to location. This finding was supported by the chi-squared test which examines the hypothesis that the samples come from the same population with respect to distribution. Again the hypothesis for each topic could not be rejected. The levels of probability were similar to those for the Kruskal-Wallis test ($\alpha = 0{\cdot}6, 0{\cdot}9, 0{\cdot}2, 0{\cdot}8, 0{\cdot}8$ respectively).

that z learners achieved a pre-score of x and a post-score of y. The diagonals are drawn to show the changes in the scores of individual learners on each topic for each treatment. Learners with scores plotted above the diagonal have improved during the experimental period.

5. The Questions to be Answered

The aim of the remainder of this Chapter is to provide from analysis of the diagnostic test results, answers to the questions defined in Chapter 6. These questions are:

1. Is it sufficient for significant learning to take place, merely to make learners aware of their weaknesses?
2. Is the use of self-help booklets a more effective learning method than a reading list?
3. Is a reading list better than no treatment?
4. Does mathematical teaching in some topics motivate students to learn in other specified topic areas?
5. Does supervised study increase learning?

6. The Measurement of Change at Mastery Level

The chief concern of this section of the research is to discover what forms of remediation enable the learners to reach the necessary mastery levels in the selected topics.

Insert 7.3 below, indicates which treatments produced a significant change in the mastery levels of the relevant groups, and Insert 7.2 shows that in each case the change was an increase in the frequency of mastery scores from pre-test to post-test.

Insert 7.3:
Changes in Mastery Levels

	T_1	T_2	T_3	T_4	T_5
H_1	*B* ****	*B* *	— NS	*L* NS	*B* ****
H_2	*B* *	*L* NS	*B* **	*B* **	— NS
H_3	— NS	— NS	— NS	— NS	— NS

B = booklet
L = reading list
— = no treatment

**** means significant at the 0·0001 level.
*** means significant at the 0·001 level.
** means significant at the 0·01 level.
* means significant at the 0·05 level
NS means not significant.

The change in the number of learners attaining mastery levels due to the treatments was examined and the conclusions were clear:[2]

1. Since Group H_3 showed no significant improvement in any of the topics, ***knowledge of their mathematical weaknesses was insufficient to improve the learners scores to mastery level.***
2. ***In every topic, the self-instructional booklets produced an increase in the number of learners achieving mastery,*** significant at least at the 0·05 level.
3. ***No such change was occasioned by the reading list.***
4. Since there was no significant improvement for groups H_1 and H_2 in the untreated topics T_3 and T_5 respectively, ***no transference of skills or motivation occurred from treated to untreated topic areas.***

It is also interesting to note that, for topics T_3 and T_5, for which the mastery level was set at a score of 5, the same significant changes occurred for learners scoring 6. That is to say that the booklets significantly increased the number of learners attaining the upper bounds of ability needed, and the reading list and pre-test alone did not.

7. The Measurement of Change at all Score Levels

None of the experimental treatments raised all the learners to mastery level, and so it was considered that deeper insight into the methods of remediation might be gained by analysis of the actual scores in addition to analysis of those of the nurses attaining mastery levels. As discussed in Chapter 2, when the pre-scores indicate that the samples come from the same population the post-scores can be directly compared for each topic, thereby minimising any effect on the analysis of change due to different initial attainment.

Three sets of results were examined.[3] These were the relationships between booklet treatment and no treatment, between reading list and no treatment, and between booklet and reading list.[4]

It was shown that the use of the appropriate booklet produces an improvement in the learners' scores significantly greater than the other treatments at least at the 0·01 level in all topics. ***The special self-instructional booklets thus provide the most effective method of remediation causing a noticeable improvement in the general level of***

---

[2] The change in the number of learners attaining mastery levels due to the treatments was examined by considering a 2 × 2 frequency table of pre- and post-mastery scores, for each group and topic, and applying the McNemar test for significance.

[3] The Mann-Whitney test was used between pairs of groups to look for significant changes in the location of the scores, and was followed by the Kolmgorov-Smirnov test for distribution.

mathematical skill in a particular topic, and a definite increase in the number of learners achieving mastery.

Although no significant change was observed at mastery level (see Insert 7.3)[2] in those learners given a library reading list, reference to Inserts 7.4 and 7.5[4] show some change did indeed occur. This can be seen in Insert 7.2 (from the distribution of scores above the diagonal) to be an improvement in both T_2 and T_4. A consideration of the comparisons of booklet and list scores in these topics, however, shows that the booklets occasioned a greater improvement, significant at the 0·001 and 0·05 level respectively. ***The reading list occasioned some improvement in the general level of achievement in the relevant mathematical skills, but significantly less than that brought about by the booklets.***

From the review of the literature in Chapter 2, it would seem that this lesser effect of the reading list could be due to many learners, in fact, not using the library. This inference seemed to be confirmed during discussion with the learners at the post-test feedback session.

The possibility of the transfer of skills and motivation to untreated areas for groups H_1 and H_2 was investigated for topics T_3 and T_5. As Inserts 7.4 and 7.5[4] show, there was no significant difference between these groups and the control group H_3 on these topics. ***The learners***

[4] Inserts 7.4 and 7.5 below give the level of significance of the difference between each treatment pair, for both statistical tests. Where booklet effects are being compared with no treatment, the significance levels are boxed in black.

Insert 7.4:
Mann-Whitney Test

Group Pair	T_1	T_2	T_3	T_4	T_5
H_1 & H_2	NS	****	*	*	****
H_1 & H_3	****	****	NS	**	****
H_2 & H_3	**	*	**	****	NS

Insert 7.5:
Kolmogorov-Smirnov Test (2-tailed)

Group Pair	T_1	T_2	T_3	T_4	T_5
H_1 & H_2	NS	***	NS	NS	****
H_1 & H_3	****	****	NS	NS	****
H_2 & H_3	**	NS	*	***	NS

**** means significant at the 0·0001 level.
*** means significant at the 0·001 level.
** means significant at the 0·01 level.
* means significant at the 0·05 level
NS means not significant.

showed no signs of incidental transfer causing improvement in the areas not given specific remedial treatment.

For topic T_1, the booklet was given to both groups H_1 and H_2. H_1 was, in addition, given specific study time in which to work at the booklet. Using the chi-squared test on the two groups for mastery and non-mastery, H_1 is not shown to be significantly better than H_2, The Mann-Whitney test on the full range of scores gives a similar result. This accords with the results of a study conducted by Loughlin *et al.* (1964), cited in Chapter 6, in which she concludes that ***enforced supervised study periods "are not the answer to student scholastic progress and increased motivation".***

8. Summary

The score frequencies of the pre- and post-tests given to three learner groups are set out in Insert 7.1. Since the samples were not normally distributed, non-parametric statistics were used to analyse all the results. **There was no significant difference between the three groups in the pre-test** when the chi-squared and Kruskal-Wallis tests were applied, and, therefore, comparisons between post-scores could be made, without making allowances for pre-existing group differences. Individual learners' score changes are displayed in Insert 7.2 and McNemar's test is used in the analysis of the numbers of learners achieving mastery levels following the various treatments. The Mann-Whitney and Kolmogorov-Smirnov tests are used to investigate score improvement below mastery level.

The five research questions can be answered as follows:

1. It is not sufficient for significant learning to take place, merely to make the learners aware of their weaknesses.
2. The self-help booklets are significantly better than any other tested treatment, both at increasing the number of learners achieving mastery level and at effecting a rise in the general standard in a particular topic.
3. The reading list is ineffective in increasing the numbers of learners reaching mastery level, but does occasion some general improvement in the treated topics.
4. Incidental skill and motivation transfer from treated to untreated topic does not occur.
5. Supervised study periods do not increase learning.

CHAPTER 8

Conclusions, Limitations and Implications of the Research into Nursing Mathematics

The intention of this research was to look at the basic mathematical skills needed by nursing learners, to consider the problems which are commonly present and to offer suggestions on remediation. To do this, it was necessary to define the mathematical skills needed by a nurse, to discover by testing learners the topics giving rise to difficulties, and to compare by means of an experiment various methods of learning open to nursing trainees. This Chapter discusses some of the conclusions which can be drawn, while bearing in mind the limitations of this research. Indications are given of the implications of the findings both for Schools of Nursing and for practising nurses. Areas in need of further research are also suggested.

1. Qualifications for Entry to Training

It became clear during this research that there exist many learners who are having problems with nursing mathematics, and that these problems do not 'go away' as a result of existing training. Various possibilities are considered.

(a) Could these difficulties be eliminated by changing the requirements for entry to Schools of Nursing? Only A-level mathematics was shown to carry the guarantee that the learner would have very few mathematical problems. Emphasis must be placed again on the point that one is considering a *real* situation, and not an *ideal* one. To insist on A-level mathematics as an entry requirement for nursing would be totally unrealistic and even undesirable. Many other qualities and skills are at least as important in a nurse and the mathematics actually required on the job is merely a small, specialised, subset of the O-level syllabus.

(b) Would a mathematics test at the time of application for admission to a School of Nursing be appropriate? Such a test does in fact exist, and was designed to be part of the alternative basic entry requirement for State Registered Nurse training. In reality the test is far more frequently used on those wishing to become State Enrolled Nurses, and it is not specifically related to the mathematics a nurse needs on the job. The major disadvantage, however, of any general mathematics test at the time of application to nurse training is that it does not test ability at entry to training and the results are thus not likely to reflect the 'forgetting' which may occur in the intervening time. (See Chapter 2: Special Learning Problems). Although not directly investigated in this research, it also seems possible that for some learners the problem is not one of basic mathematics, but of inability to see what mathematics is needed in the nursing situation (Hindam, 1960). It would thus be more appropriate to administer a diagnostic test, followed by remediation at the beginning of a nurse's training programme. Remediation must be nursing orientated to facilitate 'transfer' of any existing maths skills.

2. Motivation to Learn

Evidence has been given in Chapter 4 indicating a lack of awareness among learners of their true skills in nursing mathematics. Their judgements are likely to be based on the mathematics they remember encountering at school. One newly qualified nurse, prior to failing completely four questions on decimals, said "Oh yes, I can do decimals, we did that in primary school". Learners cannot, therefore, be relied upon to seek help when it is necessary. Even making them aware, with a diagnostic test on entry to training, is shown (Chapter 7) to be insufficient on its own to motivate them to learn. One reason for this situation may be that importance is not seen to be attached to mathematics in the Schools of Nursing. This need for remediation poses problems for tutors faced with an already full time-table for the short periods when learners are in the School. Although many agree that there is a need, they are unwilling to teach mathematics at the expense of some other aspect of nurse training.

The issuing of a relevant reading list, following a diagnostic test, would be one method of reinforcing the awareness of learners that mathematical accuracy is considered important. Unfortunately both the literature reviewed in Chapter 2 and the results of the experiment described in Chapter 7 show that the expectation that learning will occur through use of library facilities is frequently false.

Presenting learners with relevant self-help booklets, following feedback from a diagnostic test, however, produced a significant increase in the number of learners attaining mastery level in those topics, and significantly better overall results than the other remediation methods tested in the experiment (Chapter 7). In reply to Hindthorne (1980) (quoted in Chapter 2), it appears that learners will only partially accept responsibility for their own learning. They need attention focussed on their own difficulties and direct contact with specific learning materials, not merely directional pointers to suggested reading. Specially allocated study time, however, did not appear to substantially increase learning from the self-help booklets.

3. Limitations on the Conclusions

The scores needed in the experiment to achieve the set mastery levels were high, and it can be argued that a single short test does not produce sufficient evidence to establish a candidate's 'true' score (see Chapter 2). The author's counter-argument to this is that in nursing the mathematics skills are specific and vital, and in certain areas 100% mastery of the topic should be expected.

Nevertheless, one must be wary when drawing extended conclusions from the experiment. It has been demonstrated that certain self-instructional booklets produced increased learning for certain learners. Since not every learner achieved mastery, it is possible that, although self-help has been shown to be the best remedial method of those tried in the present nurse-training situation, 'second generation' self-help materials might produce even better results. It is also possible that any material presented in this concrete way (including the books used in the reading list, if they were actually given to the nurses) would stimulate interest and ability to learn. One learner commented during the post-test feedback session:

> "If you've been given it (referring to the booklet) you know you've got to learn it."

It seems probable, however, that, in fact, it is the teaching method offered by the booklets which is more conducive to learning, but this has not been conclusively proved by the experiment since it was not accurately ascertainable how many learners used the recommended library books.

4. Considerations in Specific Areas

Drug Doses. Accuracy can be crucial when calculating and administering drugs. The basic mathematical concept involved is that of ratio and proportion, and the ways of teaching this are numerous. The self-help booklets use the unitary method with safety checks and these have been shown to effect a significant increase in the number of learners reaching the set mastery levels. Another method, that of formula substitution with unit checks, as taught in Mathematics in the Ward—Drug Calculations (Pirie, 1982), has also proved effective in teaching dosage calculations. No investigations have yet been done, however, to evaluate the relative merits of alternative approaches to the problem of drug dose calculations. The extension of research to this area could also have repercussions and implications for the teaching of ratio in schools.

Graphs. This field was not dealt with satisfactorily in this study, for reasons given in Chapter 4. Nevertheless, plotting and interpreting graphs is both an important and frequent task for nurses. Further work is needed to examine the problems which are indicated by this study as existing for nursing learners. (Insert 4.1 gives 78% of the sample demonstrating difficulty in interpreting a graph.)

S.I. Units. Many years after the conversion to the S.I. of the Health Service, difficulties still exist for learners and practising nurses. It has already been suggested in earlier Chapters that contributory factors to these problems may be the reliance on conversion tables and the use of mainly Imperial measures in daily life. Both these situations inhibit the acquisition of intrinsic understanding of the 'size' of grams, millilitres, micrograms, etc. If this is the case, two stages of learning are needed:

(i) acquiring knowledge of the actual basic S.I. units and the factor of 1,000 which connects all sub-units;
(ii) gaining experience of the common quantities.

The first of these was covered by the materials used in the experiment, but the second comes only with repeated handling of substances measured and considered in S.I. units, or, failing this, from work with specially designed educational materials. Schools of Nursing can do much to help by providing continual practical or simulated experiences. The development of teaching materials in this field would undoubtedly be useful to tutors who may themselves be unfamiliar with the units.

5. Practising Nurses

The central issue of this research has been the mathematical problems of the learner, but there is no obvious reason why it should not be generalised to qualified nurses, particularly those returning to nursing after some years absence, who may well find that specifically written self-help booklets will enable them to 'brush-up' their skills, easily and without embarrassment. In particular, the utilisation of a drug doses booklet such as that used in the experiment is recommended for nurses moving to specialised wards for paediatric, diabetic or intensive care patients.

6. General Implications for the Training of Nurses

The major results of this research can briefly be summarised by answering the four questions posed in Chapter 1.

1. There now exists a taxonomy of the mathematics a nurse needs 'on the job'. (Insert 3.1.)

2. Not all learners are adequately competent in each of these mathematical fields, and the areas of common difficulty have been defined (Chapter 3).
3. Many learners are unaware of their weaknesses and their abilities.
4. Treatment by a diagnostic test and self-teaching materials seems the most effective remedy in the majority of cases.

Several immediate implications for Schools of Nursing arise from these findings.

All learners should be given, on entry into training, a diagnostic test based on the mathematics contained in the Maths-for-Nurses Taxonomy. Prompt and detailed feedback of the results to the learners would alert them to their mathematical 'weak spots' and at the same time convey the impression that certain relevant mathematical skills are considered important for nursing.

Remediation appropriate to the individual learner's needs, should then be offered. Consideration, however, must also be given to the position of the tutors in the Schools of Nursing. The restrictions imposed by present training time-tables have already been discussed, but it is also unrealistic to expect nursing tutors to be qualified mathematics teachers. It became evident during discussion with many tutors that they are worried and inhibited from teaching mathematics by their perceptions of their own lack of general mathematical skills. There is also a wide-spread misconception as to the skills which are required by today's nurse. Self-help booklets, directly related to nursing mathematics topics, have been demonstrated to be the most effective form of remediation, given the present time-table constraints. They have the added advantage of liberating tutors from a task which many do not feel adequate to perform.

7. Implications for Future Research

The various studies carried out in this research have indicated three areas in which further investigations could benefit both learners and those concerned with offering mathematical remediation.

The first of these is in the field of drug doses. Consideration of the most effective approach to the teaching of the ratio problems inherent in drug dosage calculations is recommended.

Second, the whole area of graphs in nursing needs detailed study. It is necessary both to discover the problems learners are having in drawing and interpreting, and to consider methods of remediation. It is possible that use of the graphic facilities offered by a microprocessor could be valuable here.

The final suggestion is that methods and materials be developed to enable learners to acquire a 'feel' for the S.I. Units which they will encounter as nurses. This understanding would enhance the future nurse's capacity for automatic safety checks.

In nursing, accuracy can be vital.

APPENDIX 1

Excerpt for Tutors' Topic Questionnaire

Coding

Name..

Grade..

Year of qualification

Number of years of full and part time practising nursing since qualifying

Number of years as Nursing Tutor

Mathematics	Everyday	Frequently	Occasionally	Never	Mental	Written	Calculator or Tables
1. Addition of whole numbers up to 100	1	2	3	4	7	8	9
2. Addition of whole numbers up to 1000	1	2	3	4	7	8	9
3. Subtraction of whole numbers up to 100	1	2	3	4	7	8	9
4. Subtraction of whole numbers up to 1000	1	2	3	4	7	8	9
5. Multiplication of whole numbers up to 12	1	2	3	4	7	8	9
6. Multiplication of whole numbers by multiples of 10 (e.g. $\times 40$)	1	2	3	4	7	8	9
7. Multiplication of whole numbers up to 100	1	2	3	4	7	8	9
8. Multiplication of whole numbers up to 1000	1	2	3	4	7	8	9
9. Division by whole numbers from 1 to 9	1	2	3	4	7	8	9
10. Division by whole numbers, multiples of 10	1	2	3	4	7	8	9
11. Division by whole numbers up to 100	1	2	3	4	7	8	9
12. Division by whole numbers up to 1000	1	2	3	4	7	8	9

N.B. Please check that you have circled *2* numbers for each question.

	Everyday	Frequently	Occasionally	Never	Mental	Written	Calculator or Tables
40. Conversion from fractions to decimals e.g. $12\frac{5}{16} = 12{\cdot}3125$	1	2	3	4	7	8	9
41. Conversion from decimals to fractions e.g. $7{\cdot}125 = 7\frac{1}{8}$	1	2	3	4	7	8	9
42. Approximation of answers e.g. 3·5768 is approx. $3\frac{1}{2}$	1	2	3	4			
43. Correction of answers to 3 significant figures e.g. 3·5768 = 3·58 to 3 sig. fig.	1	2	3	4			

---

44. Use of percentage as a label (no calculation involved) e.g. 2% sugar in urine	1	2	3	4	7	8	9
45. Calculations with simple percentages e.g. 10%, 25%, 50% of 80	1	2	3	4	7	8	9
46. Calculations of general percentages e.g. 43% of 26	1	2	3	4	7	8	9
47. Conversion of percentage to/from fractions e.g. $25\% = \frac{1}{4}$	1	2	3	4	7	8	9
48. Conversion of percentage to/from decimals e.g. 0·5 = 50%	1	2	3	4	7	8	9

---

49. Calculations with ratios expressed as 1 in 5	1	2	3	4	7	8	9
50. Calculations with ratios expressed as 1 to 4	1	2	3	4	7	8	9
51. Conversion of ratio to/from percentage e.g. 1 in 80 = 1·25%	1	2	3	4	7	8	9

N.B. Please check that you have circled *2* numbers for each question.

APPENDIX 2

Coding 1

Achievement Test

Section II

RESULTS

Name ....

| | | | 2 | | |

Group ....

Do all rough working on *these* sheets in the spaces left under each question.
For questions (A) to (O), (Q) and (S):
Tick the box containing the answer you think is correct *or* put your answer, if different from those given, in the empty box.
N.B. there *may* be more than one correct answer. e.g. 1/2 and 2/4 have the same value. Tick *all* correct values.
For questions (P), (R), and (T) to (W):
Answer as indicated in the question concerned.

A (1) 86 + 48 =

124	134	1214	144	170	
(carry forgotten)		(carry inserted) F	(slip)	(numbers transposed 86 + 84)	

APPENDIX 2—*contd.*

(2) 1487 + 798 =	22185	1275	2185	2285	1384		
	(carry inserted) ?F	(carries forgotten)	(carry forgotten)		(transposed numbers 487 + 897)		
B (1) 75 − 56 =	29	21	14	131	91	(19)	
	(carry forgotten)	(5 + 6 transposed (76 − 55) subtracting smallest number)	(5 of 75 lost)	(add) F	(transpose answer) F?		
(2) 1402 − 156 =	1246	1346	1244	1256	454		
		(carry forgotten)	(2 of 402 lost)	(carry forgotten) F	(1456 − 1002 i.e. subtract smallest digit and misplace 100) F		
C (1) 37 × 8 =	316	296	45	246	303		Coding 2
	sl		(add) F	(carry lost)	sl		

(2) $358 \times 125 =$	44750	1253	33650	43139	483	
		(358 716 179) F	(No carries)	(35800 7160 179) F	(add) F	
D (1) $124 \div 4 =$	301	496	031	13	48	31
	(divide from right *or* wrong columns) F	(mult) F	(Heavy working)	(divide from right) F	?	
(2) $927 \div 90 =$	10·3	13	1·3	103	130	
		(missed zero + dec point) F	(missed zero) F	(divide by 9) F	(divide by 9 + miss zero) F	
E (1) $\frac{2}{5} + \frac{4}{5} =$	$1\frac{2}{10}$	$\frac{6}{5}$	$\frac{6}{10}$	$\frac{3}{5}$	$1\frac{1}{5}$	
			(add num. & denom.) F	(add num. & denom.) F		

APPENDIX 2—*contd.*

									Coding
(2) $\frac{5}{8}+\frac{1}{2}=$	$1\frac{1}{8}$	$\frac{6}{16}$	$\frac{9}{8}$	$1\frac{2}{16}$	$\frac{6}{10}$				
		(add num. mult denom.) F			(add num. add denom.) F				
F (1) $\frac{2}{3}\times\frac{7}{12}=$	$\frac{7}{8}$	$\frac{7}{18}$	$4\frac{8}{12}$	$\frac{3}{5}$	$\frac{14}{36}$	$4\frac{2}{3}$	$1\frac{1}{4}$		3
	$\left(\frac{3\times 7}{2\times 12}\right)$ F		$\left(\frac{8\times 7}{12}\right)$ F	$\left(\frac{2+7}{3+12}\right)$ F		$\left(\frac{8\times 7}{12}\right)$ F	$\left(\frac{8+7}{12}\right)$ F		
(2) $2\frac{1}{2}\times\frac{1}{20}=$	$\frac{5}{40}$	$2\frac{1}{40}$	$\frac{3}{40}$	$\frac{1}{8}$	$\frac{1}{20}$	1	$2\frac{1}{20}$		
		$(2(\frac{1}{2}\times\frac{1}{20}))$ F	$(\frac{3}{2}\times\frac{1}{20})$ F		$(8\frac{1}{2}\times 20)$ F	$\left(2\times\frac{10\times 1}{20}\right)$ F	$\left(2\times\frac{1+1}{2\times 20}\right)$ F		
G (1) $1{\cdot}5+3{\cdot}4=$	4·28	0·328	5·8	4·9	0·428				
	?	F	$\left(\begin{matrix}1{\cdot}5+4{\cdot}3\\(3{\cdot}4)\end{matrix}\right)$		?F				

							Coding
(2) 2·5+0·78 =	10·4	3·28	2·28	328	2·578		
	(2·5+7·8 = 10·4!) F		(missed carry)	(no dec. point) F	(+0·078) F?		
H (1) 0·35−0·07 =	0·42	0·18	0·028	0·38	28	0·28	
	(add) F	(miscarry carry)	(dec. pt.) F	(lost carry)	(no dec. point) F		
(2) 0·035−0·0125 =	0·225	0·0475	0·0235	0·3375	0·0225		
	(dec. pt.) F	(add) F	(lost carry)	(0·35−) F			
I (1) 0·24×5 =	120	1·2	5·120	6·20	1·20		4
	(dec. pl.) F		(5×0 = 5 +0·120) F	(5×0 = 5) F			

APPENDIX 2—*contd.*

(2) 0·071 × 145 =	10·295	0·3905	0·10295	10·085	11·895	
		(misalign 355 2840 71 3905) F	(dec. pt.) F	(! 145 284 71 10·085) (change mult method in middle)	?	
J (1) 0·25 ÷ 5 =	0·5	0·20	5	0·05	20	
	(dec. pt.) F	subtract or 5 ÷ 25	(dec. pt.) F		(5 ÷ 0·25) F	
(2) 3·28 ÷ 40 =	0·0802	0·82	13·12	0·0082	12·19	
	(0802 4)328 32 08)	(dec. pt.) F	(mult) F	(dec. pt.) F	(40 ÷ 3·28) F	

K (1) $2{\cdot}03 \div 0{\cdot}5 =$

4·06	1·015	4·6	406	2·06	0·406	0·2006	0·2413	
	(mult) F	(lost zero)	(dec. pt.) F	(2 + 0·03 ÷ 5 only ÷ dec. part by 0·5)	(dec. pt.) F	only ÷ dec. part by 0·5 F	(0·5 ÷ 2·03) NOT F (see J(2) above)	

L (1) Express $\frac{42}{1000}$ as a decimal

0·0042	0·42	23·80	0·042	4·2	
(dec. pt.) F	(dec. pt.) F	($\frac{1000}{42}$) F		(dec. pt.) F	

(2) Express $\frac{3}{8}$ as a decimal

3·75	0·375	0·38	2·66	0·37	
(dec. pt.) F		(corrected)	($\frac{8}{3}$) F	(truncated)	

M (1) Express 3·75 as a fraction

$\frac{3}{8}$	$3\frac{1}{4}$	$\frac{9}{4}$	$\frac{13}{4}$	$\frac{6}{4}$	($3\frac{3}{4}$)
(From L(2)?) F	($0{\cdot}75 = \frac{1}{4}$)	$\left(\frac{3 \times 3}{4}\right)$ F	($0{\cdot}75 = \frac{1}{4}$)	$\left(\frac{3 + 3}{4}\right)$ F	

Coding 5

APPENDIX 2—*contd.*

N (1) What is 2% of 350?

70	1·75	7	5	14	
(dec. pt.)	(½%)		(sl. (5 × 5 = 35))	(2% × 2)	

O (1) 80 ml of solution has been made up in the ratio 1 to 4. How many ml of drug does it contain?

16	20	5	64	60	
	('in') F	(1 + 4) F	(water)	(water 'in') F	

(2) A drug solution is available as 5 mg in 400 ml. How much of the solution is needed if 15 mg of pure drug are to be used?

20	6000	1200	80	20·6	
(15 + 5) F	(400 × 15) F		(400 ÷ 5) F	(400 ÷ 15) F	(1185 = water)

P (1) 1·5 kg =	g	(1500)
(2) 456 micrograms =	mg	(0·456)
(3) 180 mm =	m	(0·18)
(4) 4 1 =	ml	(4000)
(5) Given 1 Calorie = 4184 joules,	then 1 Calorie =	(Kilojoules 4·184)
(6)	1 Calorie =	(Megajoules 0·004184)

Q (1) Given that amount needed $= \dfrac{\text{strength wanted}}{\text{strength available}}$,

how many ml of solution strength 600 μg per ml are needed if you want 1 ml of strength 400 μg per ml.

1·5	4	$\frac{2}{3}$	24	10	(0·67)
$\left(\frac{600}{400}\right)$ F	$\left(\frac{400\ \mu g =}{4\ ml}\right)$ F		(6×4) F	$(6+4)$ F	

(2) Daily fluid requirement in ml, for a baby, is given as 150 × weight in kg. How much does a baby aged 10 weeks and weighing 4·1 kg need?

41	615	61·5	600	15	
$(4{\cdot}1 \times 10)$ F		$\left(\frac{150 \times 4{\cdot}1}{10}\right)$ F	(150×4)	$\left(\frac{150}{100}\right)$ F	

R (1) Use the given table to find:

10 stone 5 lb. =	kg (65·77)
119 lb. =	kg (53·98)
69 kg. =	stone lb (10st 12lb) (to nearest lb)
8 kg =	lb (to nearest lb) (18 lbs)

APPENDIX 2—*contd.*

Coding 7

S (1) 2×10^6 =

20^6	10^{12}	120	2 000 000	10^8	200 000	64	640	
$((2 \times 10)^6)$ F	$(10^{(2 \times 6)})$ F	$(2 \times 6 \times 10)$ F		$(10^{(6+2)})$ F	(2×10^5) F	(2^6) F	$(2^6 \times 10)$ F	

T (1) Put in order of size, smallest first, 0·7, 0·23, 0·015, 0·009, 0·205.

(0·009)	(0·015)	(0·205)	(0·23)	(0·7)

Coding 8

U (1) A child from a primitive African tribe is weighed on the 1st of each month at a clinic and the following series of results are recorded:

7·6 kg, 7·8 kg, 7·6 kg, 7·85 kg, 7·5 kg, 6·15 kg, 6·7 kg, 7·75 kg, 7·5 kg, 7 kg, 6·6 kg, 7·65 kg.

Record these weights in the table given.

V (1) Plot the weights on a graph.

W (1) Does the child lose weight at any time?
If so, during which months?

(Feb	April	May	Aug	Sept	Oct)
2	4	5	8	9	10

(2) Judging by the graph, has the child made satisfactory growth over the year?
(No)

X (1) Add together 0·25, −0·125 and 1·7.

1·925	−2·075	1·835	0·70	0·825	1·825
(−0·025)	(0·25 + 0·125 + 1·7 = 2·075 = −2·075 F)	(lost carry)	(−1·25)	(0·7)	

APPENDIX 3

Section I

Excerpt from the Self-assessment Survey

1. Name...

| | | | 1 | | | Group..

| 0 |

2. Grade:

| 1 | SRN

| 2 | SEN

3. Year

| 1 | 1st year

| 2 | 2nd year

| 3 | 3rd year

4. Maths qualifications:

| 1 | A levels

| 2 | O levels or CSE grade 1

3 CSE other grades

Another maths qualification; state what:............................

4 No maths qualifications

5. Other relevant qualifications:

1 A level

2 O level or CSE grade 1

3 CSE other grades

Other qualifications; state what..

4 No other relevant qualification

0

continued

In the next part of this section you are asked to rate the difficulty you would find in doing certain mathematics.

Easy means:	could do it in my head might need a scrap of paper sure of how to do it confident the answer will be right
Fairly easy means:	could probably do it given time would definitely need paper or tables reasonably sure I know how to do it fairly confident the answer would be right
Difficult means:	would need some help would need a calculator not quite sure how to do it would need to check with someone
Impossible means:	could not do it would get someone else to do it for me have never understood this don't know how to begin

Example

Easy	Fairly easy	Difficult	Impossible	
				(z) Conversion of units e.g. Turn $10\frac{1}{2}$ stone to kg.

Tick 'Fairly Easy' if you could do it using tables.
Tick 'Difficult' if you would need someone to help you.

	Easy	Fairly Easy	Difficult	Impossible	*Topics*
(a)	1	2	3	4	(a) Addition of whole numbers e.g. $1254+329$
(b)	1	2	3	4	(b) Subtraction of whole numbers e.g. $1360-177$

(c)	1	2	3	4	(c) Multiplication of whole numbers e.g. 262×135
(d)	1	2	3	4	(d) Division of whole numbers e.g. $294 \div 70$
(e)	1	2	3	4	(e) Addition of fractions e.g. $\frac{3}{5} + \frac{3}{20}$
(f)	1	2	3	4	(f) Multiplication of fractions e.g. $3\frac{4}{7} \times \frac{2}{5}$
(g)	1	2	3	4	(g) Addition of decimals e.g. $0{\cdot}26 + 3{\cdot}15$
(h)	1	2	3	4	(h) Subtraction of decimals e.g. $0{\cdot}25 - 0{\cdot}065$
(i)	1	2	3	4	(i) Multiplication of decimals e.g. $0{\cdot}725 \times 132$
(j)	1	2	3	4	(j) Division of decimals e.g. $26{\cdot}43 \div 30$
(k)	1	2	3	4	(k) Division by decimals e.g. $4{\cdot}9 \div 0{\cdot}8$
(l)	1	2	3	4	(l) Turning fractions to decimals e.g. $\frac{5}{8} = (0{\cdot}625)$

APPENDIX 4

Excerpt from the Self-instructional Booklets

DRUG DOSES

INTRODUCTION

This booklet is one of a series of self-help books which have been written specifically for nurses and nursing learners.

The series is designed to help you with your particular difficulties in the sort of mathematics you will need as a nurse.

You will need pencil and paper.

The book is divided into sections with explanations and examples on the right-hand page, followed by a few straightforward questions for you to work on the left-hand page. Answer these questions *on paper* (not in the book) and then turn to the back to check your answers. If you have *ALL* your answers correct turn on to the next page. If not, go back over the text carefully and then try the check test again.

There are 2 revision tests, one about half way through the topic and one at the end. The answers to these questions are given with page references, so that you can check again any area where you have made mistakes.

From time to time you will see sections of work inside square brackets, e.g. [Reminder: the decimals you have been using . . .] This means that the section is not direct teaching on the booklet topic, but is a quick revision of some piece of knowledge needed for the next section of the topic.

Do not try to do more than 3 or 4 sections and their checks without a break. Five or ten minutes (or even 2 days!) rest will help to fix what you have already learned and restore your powers of concentration. If you feel that you are floundering or getting bogged down, STOP. Go away and come back later when you are feeling calmer and ready to try again.

This booklet shows you a method of calculating *any* drug dose, however it is prescribed or packaged. If you always follow this method (which includes a safety check) you will be a safe and competent nurse when handling drugs.

Since it is hoped that many learners will use this booklet during their initial training block, some of the medical "jargon" used when writing prescriptions (I.V., q.i.d., etc.) has been omitted from the worked examples to avoid confusion and allow the learner to concentrate on the *calculations* involved in drug doses. A reference list of common abbreviations is given at the end of the booklet.

DRUG DOSES

Giving patients medicine is one part of a nurse's work which everyone knows about. Most people, too, are well aware of the dangers of overdoses. Tragic mistakes resulting in death are given wide coverage by the press and these mistakes are usually mathematical mistakes. Every nurse needs to be 100% accurate every time a dose of medicine is given.

Fortunately calculating drug doses can be simple, as you will see.

You may well meet, or even have already met, several different ways of calculating a drug dose. Books and tutors use various formulae all of which eventually produce the right answer for the drug being administered.

In this booklet you will learn that there is one, very simple formula which will always work.

Why is there any problem at all, since it is the doctor who prescribes the dose that a patient will be given? Surely all the nurse has to do is just give it? The problem is that the medicament prescribed by a doctor may not be packaged in the precise dose which he wants to administer.

Consider a simple example. The doctor prescribes a dose of 8 mg of Nicoumalone (an anti-coagulant) for a patient being treated for thrombosis. This drug is supplied in 4 mg tablets. The nurse must therefore work out how many tablets the patient should be given. 2 tablets—easy!

Stop and think how you worked that out:

The dose prescribed was 8 mg

The dose per pill was 4 mg

$$\text{So the number of pills to be given} = \frac{\text{the dose prescribed}}{\text{the dose per pill}} = \frac{8}{4} = 2$$

Look at another example:

The doctor prescribes 75 mg of amitriptyline for a patient suffering from depression.

Amitriptyline comes in 25 mg pills.

Dose prescribed = 75 mg

Dose per pill = 25 mg

$$\text{So number of pills} = \frac{\text{dose prescribed}}{\text{dose per pill}} = \frac{75}{25} = 3.$$

Accuracy in drug administration is vital. Mistakes are easily made. *Always look at the result of your calculations and think "Is that a sensible answer?"*

Look at the examples on this page. Even though you are not familiar with the particular drugs being used you can consider 2 or 3 pills as a reasonable dose. 8 or 10 would not be a reasonable dose so you would need to re-check your working.

Pills

Check (1)

A. A pain killer is prescribed for a woman in labour in a single dose of 50 mg. The capsules contain 25 mg of the drug each. How many capsules should she be given?

B. Aspirin is dispensed in 300 mg pills. How many pills are needed for a dose of 900 mg?

C. How many pills are needed each day for a dose of 600 mg, three times a day?

D. The dose of 150 mg of aspirin is recommended for a five year old child. How many pills should be given?

E. Penicillin is dispensed in 250 mg pills. How many pills are needed to give a child a dose of 125 mg?

So now we have a formula which copes with pills. What about liquid medicines?

A doctor prescribes 10 mg of codeine as a cough depressant. Codeine is dispensed as 5 mg of codeine per 5 ml spoonful of linctus.

Dose prescribed = 10 mg
Dose per spoonful = 5 mg

So the patient will need 2 spoonfuls of linctus.

Is this a reasonable answer? Yes, 2 spoonfuls is a quantity acceptable to a patient.

How did we work that out? Is there a formula being used here like the pill formula?

$$\text{Yes. Number of teaspoonfuls} = \frac{\text{Dose prescribed}}{\text{Dose per 5 ml spoonful}} = \frac{10}{5} = 2.$$

Example

A doctor prescribes 25 mg of a drug to be given by injection. It is a drug dispensed in a solution of strength 50 mg per ml.

How many ml should the nurse give?

Dose prescribed = 25 mg
Dose per ml = 50 mg

$$\text{Number of ml to be given} = \frac{\text{Dose prescribed}}{\text{Dose per ml}} = \frac{25}{50} = \frac{1}{2} = 0{\cdot}5 \text{ ml}.$$

Reasonable answer? Yes, 0·5 ml is a common quantity to inject.

Liquids

How can you check whether your calculation has been correct?

Medicines are manufactured and packed in a form which will make a dose both palatable to the patient (e.g. not more than 3 or 4 spoonfuls) and easy to administer by the nurse (e.g. not in such concentrated form that the nurse needs to give $\frac{1}{5}$ of a pill). All drugs are now dispensed in metric quantities, most commonly mg and ml. The "teaspoonful" has been replaced by the "5-ml medicine spoon" which is a little larger.

Hints to remember, therefore, when checking your calculations (even for unfamiliar drugs) are:

(i) 15 to 20 ml (3 to 4 medicine spoonfuls) are likely to be the maximum dose of a liquid medicament, taken orally.
(ii) 3 or 4 pills or capsules are likely to be the maximum dose of solid medicaments.
(iii) Injection quantities normally range between 0·25 ml and 2 ml.
(iv) A child's dose is almost always less than the adult standard dose. (The result "$\frac{1}{2}$ an aspirin" was a reasonable answer for the dose for a child in check 1).

As you become more experienced you will remember the normal quantities prescribed for the drugs in common use and this will obviously make it easy to check your dose calculations.

BUT familiar or unfamiliar, you must *ALWAYS CHECK* your answers for "unreasonableness".

"Reasonableness" checks

Check (2)
Omnopon (an injection containing opium) comes in an ampule containing 20 mg in 1 ml.

A. How many ml should be injected if 10 mg are prescribed?
B. How many ml are to be injected if 15 mg are prescribed?
Comment on your answers.

C. Digoxin is a drug used in connection with the heart. A stock bottle contains elixir with 0·05 mg per ml. If the prescription is 0·5 mg, how much elixir should be given?
D. A nurse reads a prescription for 2·5 mg of digoxin. How much elixir should she give?
Comment on your answers.

E. The stock bottle of sulphadimidine, used to arrest the growth of bacteria, contains 100 mg per ml. The prescription reads 300 mg as an initial dose. How many ml should be given?
F. A nurse takes the stock bottle of ampillicin 25 g per ml to give an oral dose of 0·5 g. How many ml should she give?
Comment on your answers.

So far we have three formulae for drug calculations:

(i) Number of pills $= \dfrac{\text{Dose prescribed}}{\text{Dose per pill}}$

(ii) Number of 5 ml spoonfuls $= \dfrac{\text{Dose prescribed}}{\text{Dose per 5 ml spoonful}}$

(iii) Number of ml $= \dfrac{\text{Dose prescribed}}{\text{Dose per ml}}$

BUT you were promised *one* formula which always works!

We can in fact make a general formula which does cover all these separate cases.
Consider:

$$\text{Number of “measures” to be given} = \frac{\text{Dose prescribed}}{\text{Dose per “measure”}}$$

If the "measure" is a pill we have formula (i)
If the "measure" is a millilitre we have formula (iii) etc.
A "measure" need not always be pills, spoonfuls or ml.

Problem

A patient needs 160 calories. A boiled egg contains 80 calories.
How many eggs should he have for breakfast?
It is the "How much . . ." or "How many . . ." part of the problem which gives you what your "measure" is.

So if we say the "measure" is an egg, we have

$$\text{Number of eggs} = \frac{\text{Dose prescribed}}{\text{Dose per egg}} = \frac{160}{80} = 2 \text{ (Correct!)}$$

LEARN THIS FORMULA:

$$\boxed{\text{Number of “measures” to be given} = \frac{\text{Dose prescribed}}{\text{Dose per “measure”}}}$$

The formula

Check (3)

A. What is the drug formula which must be indelibly written on your heart?
B. Having done your calculation from the formula, what next?

CHECK THESE ANSWERS BEFORE YOU GO ON

TAKE A BREAK NOW

[Reminder:
There are 1000 micrograms in 1 milligram.
The *typed* abbreviation for microgram is μ.
NEVER write μg yourself, always write microgram in full, because it is easy to misread μg as mg.]

In all the examples we have looked at, the units for the dose prescribed and for the dose per "measure" have been the same. e.g. Doctor prescribed 75 *mg* of amitryptyline and it comes in 25 *mg* pills e.g. Doctor prescribed in 10 *mg* codeine and this is dispensed as *5 mg* per 5 ml-spoon.

What happens if the doctor prescribes an injection 200 micrograms of drug and the stock bottle contains 1 milligram per ml?

Here we have Dose prescribed in micrograms and
Dose per "measure" in milligrams.

Before you use the golden formula you must make sure that the two dose values are in the same unit. If they are not, as in this case, you must convert the dose prescribed to the same units as the dose per "measure".*

Here we have
'Dose-per-measure' unit = *mg* (1 mg per ml)
Dose prescribed = 200 μg = 0·2 *mg*

The formula then gives: Number of "measures" (ml) to be given $= \frac{0{\cdot}2}{1} = 0{\cdot}2$.

The injection is 0·2 ml, which is reasonable!

* Strictly speaking, it does not matter what units you use as long as they are the same for both dose values. BUT the arithmetic is *usually easier* if you convert to the units of the dose per "measure".

Converting the units

APPENDIX 5

Excerpt from the Diagnostic Test

INTRODUCTORY BLOCK TEST

Actual question used:

1. Nicoumalone, an anti-coagulant, comes in 4 mg tablets. A doctor prescribes 10 mg for a patient with a thrombosis. How many pills must the patient have?

Generalised Item Specification:

All questions of the form:
"Prescription is a units 1, available as b units 2, in c units 3"
where $c = 1$, *unit 3 = tablet, units 1 = units 2,* $\frac{b}{a}$ *integer or integer +* $\frac{1}{2}$

2. A patient needs 25 mg of a drug, injected every *4* hours. The drug is dispensed in ampoules containing 50 mg per ml. How many ampoules are used for each injection?

$c = 1$, *unit 3 = 1 ampoule (containing 1 ml)*
unit 1 = unit 2
$a < b$
Some irrelevant number in the question

3. Omnopon, an opium injection, is available as a 20 mg per ml solution. How many ml will be given to a patient prescribed 5 mg?

$c = 1$, *unit 3 = ml*
unit 1 = unit 2
$a = b$

4. A doctor prescribes a dose of 30 units of soluble insulin. The available stock is of strength 20 units/ml. How many ml will the patient be given?

$c = 1$, *unit 3 = ml*
unit 1 = unit 2 = "unit"
Question related to insulin
$a > b$

5. 12 mg of Valergan, an oral pre-medication, are to be given to a child. Valergan syrup is available in 30 mg per 5 ml strength. How much of the syrup must the child have?

c ≠ 1, unit 3 = ml
unit 1 = unit 2
a ≠ b

6. 5 ml of syrup contain 500 micrograms of a drug. How much syrup does a patient need to be given, to get 0·5 mg of the drug?

c ≠ 1, unit 3 = ml
unit 1 ≠ unit 2

APPENDIX 6

Reading List

S.I. Units

Recommended Reading

There are many different publications which contain a chapter or article on S.I. Units.

There are two particular books which have been written directly for nurses and which have a chapter on S.I. Units.

These are:

JEFFERIES, P. M. (1978). *Mathematics in Nursing, fifth edition.* London, Baillière Tindall, Chapter 9.

WATCHORN, G. W. (1976). *Medical Calculations for Nurses, second edition.* London, Faber and Faber, Chapter 1.

Formulae

Recommended Reading

There are many different publications which contain a chapter or article on working with formulae.

There are two particular books which have been written directly for nurses and which contain some material on formulae.

These are:

JEFFERIES, P. M. (1978). *Mathematics in Nursing, fifth edition,* London, Baillière Tindall, p. 104, p. 111–117, p. 133–135.

WATCHORN, G. W. (1976). *Medical Calculations for Nurses, second edition,* London, Faber and Faber, p. 28–29, p. 54–55.

References

ADELMAN, C. and WALKER, R. (1975). Developing pictures for other frames: action research and case study'. Chapter 12. In: *Frontiers of Classroom Research,* G. Chanan and S. Delamont, NFER.

AIRASIAN, P. W. (1972). An application of mastery learning strategy. *Psychology in the Schools,* Vol. 9, No. 2, pp. 130–34.

ANDERSON, E. M. and VERVOREN, T. M. (1976). *Workbook of Solution and Dosage of Drugs including Arithmetic. (10th Edition).* St Louis, Mosby.

ANDERTON, P. and BIGG, P. H. (1972). *Changing to the Metric System N.P.L. (4th Edition).* HMSO.

APPLE, J. L. (1976). The classification of medication errors. *Supervisory Nurse* Vol. 7, December, pp. 23–25, 28–29.

AVENT, C. (1977). Changing aspirations and values of young people. *Coombe Lodge Reports,* Vol. 9, No. 16, pp. 568–571.

AUSUBEL, D. P. (1968). *Educational Psychology: a cognitive view.* New York, Holt Rinehart and Winston.

BADGER, M. E. (1981). Why aren't girls better at maths? A review of research. *Educational Research,* Vol. 24, November, No. 1.

BAILEY, R. E. (1980). *Multiple Choice Questions, Book 3, Pharmacology for Nurses.* London, Baillière Tindall.

BARKER, K. N. and McCONNELL, W. E. (1962). How to detect medication errors. *The Modern Hospital,* Vol. 99, No. 1, pp. 95–106.

BARON, D. N. (1974) Contemporary themes: S.I. Units. *British Medical Journal,* November, pp. 509–512.

BATTY, G. R. (1975). The dilemma of the unit-dose pharmacy system. *Hospital Administration in Canada,* Vol. 17, No. 11 and 12, pp. 49–50.

BENT, H. (1974). No easy way: experience with a modified Keller physical chemistry course. *Journal of Chemical Education,* Vol. 51, October, pp. 661–4.

BIRKHALTER, P. (1972). Medication errors: Let's eliminate them. *Supervisory Nurse,* Vol. 3, pp. 58–62.

BLATCHLEY, M. E. (1978). Effects of self-study on achievement in a medical-surgical nursing course. *Nursing Outlook,* Vol. 26, July, pp. 444–7.

BLOCK, J. H. (1971). *Mastery Learning.* New York, Holt Rinehart and Winston.

BLOOM, B. S., HASTINGS, J. T. and MADUS, G. F. (1971). *Handbook on Formative and Sumative Evaluation of Student Learning.* New York, McGraw Hill.

BOND, J. (1974). The construction of a scale to measure nurses' attitudes. *International Journal of Nursing Studies,* Vol. 11, pp. 75–84.

BOND, S. (1980). Sources and resources. *Nursing Times,* Vol. 76, June, pp. 1106–9.

BOORER, D. (1969). Nurses who do not read. *Nursing Times,* Vol. 65, July, pp. 984–5.

Bormuth, J. R. (1970). *On the Theory of Achievement Test Items*. Chicago, University of Chicago Press.

Bouchard, J. (1980). Contract learning. *Canadian Nurse*, Vol. 76, January, pp. 44–48.

Brown, G. C. (1979). Medication errors: a case study. *Hospitals*, Vol. 53, October, pp. 61–62, 65.

Budd, R. (1971). We changed to unit-dose system. *Nursing Outlook*, Vol. 19, February, pp. 116–117.

Burke, R. J. (1969). Some preliminary data on the use of self-evaluation and peer ratings in assigning university course grades. *Journal of Educational Research*, Vol. 62, No. 10, pp. 444–5.

Button, D. (1966). *Maths for Nurses, a Course for Pre-Nursing Students. (3rd Edition)*. London, Faber.

Campbell, D. T. and Stanley, J. C. (1967). Experimental and quasi-experimental designs for research on teaching. *Handbook of Research on Teaching*, (ed. N. L. Gage), Chicago, Rand McNally, (Chapter 5, pp. 171–247).

Carr, J. J., McElroy, N. L. and Carr, B. L. (1976). How to solve dosage problems in one easy lesson. *American Journal of Nursing*, Vol. 76, December, pp. 1934–1937.

Carroll, J. B. (1963). A model of school learning. *Teachers' College Record*, Vol. 64, pp. 723–733.

Cockcroft, W. H. (1982). Report of a Government Committee of Inquiry into the Teaching and Learning of Mathematics in Secondary Schools. *Mathematics Counts*. (Chairman: W. H. Cockcroft.) London, HMSO.

Coffey, L. L. (1978). Independent/individualised learning. *Nursing Forum*, Vol. 17, pp. 84–95.

Conners, C. K. and Eisenberg, L. (1966). *The Effect of Teacher Behaviour on Verbal Intelligence in Operation Headstart Children*. Baltimore, School of Medicine, Johns Hopkins University.

Cook, T. D. and Campbell, D. T. (1979). *Quasi-Experimentation: Design and Analysis*. Chicago, Rand McNally.

Cornell, F. G., Lindvall, C. M. and Saupe, J. L. (1952). *An Exploratory Measurement of Individualities of Schools and Classrooms*. Bureau of Educational Research, College of Education, University of Illinois.

Cowan, J. (1975). The ability to appraise one's own work. *Higher Education Bulletin*, Vol. 3, No. 2, pp. 127–128.

Cronbach, L. J. and Furby, L. (1970). How we should measure change—or should we? *Psychological Bulletin*, Vol. 74, No. 1, pp. 68–80.

Cronbach, L. J. and Glaser, G. C. (1965). *Psychological Tests and Personnel Decisions. (2nd Edition.)* Urbana Illinois, University of Illinois Press.

Crooks, J., Clark, C. G., Caie, H. B. and Mawson, W. B. (1965). Prescribing and administration of drugs in hospital. *Lancet*, Vol. 1, pp. 373–378.

Daines, J. M. (1978). Self-evaluation of academic performance in a continuously assessed course of study. *Research Intelligence*, Vol. 4, No. 1, pp. 24–26.

Davis, B. (1980). Information please! *Nursing Times*, Vol. 76, June, p. 1109.

Department of Education and Science. (1979). *Aspects of Secondary Education in England*. London, HMSO.

Department of Education and Science. (1980). *Aspects of Supplementary Information on Mathematics.* London, HMSO.

Department of Health and Social Security. (1980). *Directory of Schools of Nursing.* HMSO.

Dexter, P. and Applegate, M. (1980). How to solve a math problem. *Journal of Nursing Education.* Vol. 19, No. 2, February, pp. 49–53.

Dison, N. (1980). *Simplified Drug and Solution for Nurses, including Arithmetic, 7th Edition.* St Louis, Mosby.

Donohue, J. D., Litz, K. A. and Scott, S. A. (1976). PSI: an innovative approach to teaching nursing technologies. *Journal of Nursing Education,* Vol. 15, p. 7–12.

Dunn, B. H. and Cherry, A. C. (1980). A priority for the '80s; self-assessment and recertification. *Paediatric Nursing,* Vol. 6, p. 46.

Ebel, R. L. (1969). Expected reliability as a function of choices per item. *Educational and Psychological Measurement,* Vol. 29, pp. 565–570.

Eisenbach, R. (1977). *Calculating and Administering Medications; Self-instruction.* Philadelphia, F. A. Davis Co.

Emerson, D. W. (1975). Teaching organic chemistry by a modified Keller plan. *Journal of Chemical Education,* Vol. 52, pp. 228–9.

Emmerich, W. (1968). Personality development and concepts of structure. *Child Development,* Vol. 39, pp. 671–690.

Feldt, L. S. (1958). A comparison of the precision of 3 experimental designs employing a concomitant variable. *Psychometrika,* Vol. 23, No. 4, pp. 335–353.

Ferster, M. B. (1961). *Arithmetic for Nurses: programmed for class and home study.* New York, Springer.

Fisher, R. A. (1951). *The Design of Experiments, 6th Edition.* New York, Hafner.

Fisher, R. F. and Strank, R. A. (1971). Investigation into reading habits of qualified nurses. *Nursing Times,* Vol. 67, No. 8, pp. 245–7.

Fitch, E. G., Larson, M. A and Mooney, M. P. (1977). *Basic Arithmetic Review and Drug Therapy.* New York, Macmillan.

Fitton, J. M. (1980). Why don't nurses read? *Nursing Times,* Vol. 76, July, pp. 1159–60.

Fitzgerald, A. (1976). School maths and the requirements of industry. *The Vocational Aspect of Education.* (Bolton College of Technology), Vol. 28, No. 70, pp. 43–49.

Fitzgerald, A. (1978). Pupils' performances on industrial selection tests in relation to their mathematical backgrounds. *Educational Research,* Vol. 20, No. 2, pp. 122–129.

Fitzgerald, A. (1979). Measuring the arithmetical competence of pupils in relation to employment. *Vocational Aspect of Education* (Bolton College of Technology), Vol. 31, No. 78, April, pp. 9–21.

Flanders, N. A. (1970). *Analysing Teaching Behaviour.* Reading, Massachusetts, Addison Wesley.

Ford, P. M. and Ellis, S. (1973). Unit dose drug distribution at ward level (experiment at Hospital for Women at Leeds). *Nursing Times,* Vol. 69, September, pp. 1262–65.

Frost, D. (1972). Drug mistakes in hospitals—review of the prescription and administration of medicines in hospitals, by E. A. Hedley, D. C. Moir, and R. D. Weir, Waverley Press, Aberdeen. *Nursing Times,* Vol. 68, August, pp. 978–979.

GAGE, N. L. and BERLINER, D. C. (1979). *Educational Psychology, 2nd Edition.* Chicago, Rand McNally.

GENTINE, M. (1980). Methods of teaching revisited. Self-learning packages. *Journal of Continuing Education in Nursing,* Vol. 11, May, pp. 57–59.

GILBERT, M. F. (1973). *Arithmetic for Nurses, 2nd Edition.* New York, Springer.

GILBERT, T. F. (1978). *Human Competence.* New York, McGraw Hill.

GILLIES, D. A. and ALYN, I. B. (1980). *Saunders Test for Self-evaluation of Nursing Competence, 4th Edition.* Philadelphia, Saunders.

GLASER, R. and NITKO, A. (1971). Measurement in learning and instruction. In: R. L. Thorndike (ed.) *Educational Measurement, 2nd Edition.* Washington, American Council on Education, pp. 625–670.

GLEN, J. and MCCAUGHERTY, D. (1981). *S.I. Units for Nurses.* London, Harper and Row.

GOODMAN, L. A. (1954). Kolmogorov-Smirnov tests for psychological research. *Psychological Bulletin,* Vol. 51, No. 2, pp. 160–168.

GOOSTRAY, S. (1963). *Maths and Measurements in Nursing Practice, 3rd Edition.* New York, Macmillan.

GRONLUND, N. E. (1968a). *Constructing Achievement Tests.* Englewood Cliffs, Prentice-Hall Inc.

GRONLUND, N. E. (1968b). *Readings in Measurement and Evaluation.* London, Macmillan.

GRONLUND, N. E. (1976). *Measurement and Evaluation in Teaching, 3rd Edition.* London, Macmillan.

GUILDFORD, J. P. and FRUCHTER, B. (1978). *Fundamental Statistics in Psychology and Education, 6th Edition.* New York, McGraw Hill.

HAMBLETON, R. K. and NOVICK, M. R. (1973). Towards an integration of theory and method for criterion-referenced tests. *Journal of Educational Measurement,* Vol. 10, pp. 159–170.

HARRIS, C. W. (ed.) (1967) *Problems in Measuring Change,* Madison, University of Wisconsin Press.

HARRIS, M. and LIGVORI, R. (1974). Some effects of a personalised system of instruction in teaching college mathematics: mastery learning. *Journal of Educational Research,* Vol. 68, pp. 62–6.

HART, L. K. (1969 and 1981). *The Arithmetic of Dosages and Solutions: a programmed presentation, 2nd and 5th Editions.* St Louis, Mosby.

HEATH, J. (1979). A new kind of nurse 1. Tomorrow's approach to learning. *Nursing Mirror.* Vol. 149, August, pp. 22–23.

HENDERSON, V. (1977). *Awareness of Library Resorces.* Pamphlet published by American Nursing Association (G-125), pp. 1–15.

HERMAN, G. D. (1976). Self-pacing and occupational curriculum development. *The Vocational Aspect of Education* (Bolton College of Technology), Vol. 28, No. 70, pp. 67–72.

HICKS, C. (1981). A case for action. *Nursing Times,* Vol. 77, May, p. 847.

HINDAM, Y. H. (1960). *The Effect of Familiar and Unfamiliar Settings on Problem Solving in Maths.* The Education Department, University of Birmingham.

HINDTHORNE, R. (1980). Methods of teaching revisited: self-instructional modules. *Journal of Continuing Education in Nursing,* Vol. 11, July, pp. 37–39.

HITCH, G. J. (1978). The numerical abilities of industrial trainee apprentices. *Journal of Occupational Psychology,* Vol. 51, pp. 163–176.

HIVELY, W., PATTERSON, H. L. and PAGE, S. A. (1968). A universe defined system of arithmetic achievement tests. *Journal of Educational Measurement,* Vol. 5, pp. 275–290.

HOGSTEL, M. O. (1976). A system for personalised instruction. *Nursing Outlook,* Vol. 24, February, pp. 110–114.

HOWIE, E. (1981). *Mathematical Requirements of Commerce.* Tayside Region Advisory Committee.

HUCKABAY, L. and ARNDT, G. (1976). Effects of acquisition of knowledge on self-evaluation. *Nursing Research,* Vol. 25, July, pp. 244–251.

HUCKABAY, L. M. D. (1981). The effects of modularized instruction and traditional teaching techniques on cognitive learning and affective behaviours of student nurses. *Advances in Nursing Science,* April, pp. 67–83.

HULL, E. J., ISAACS, B. J. and MARSON, S. N. (1977). *The Arithmetic of Drug Dosage.* London, Hodder and Stoughton.

I.M.A. (1974–76). *Maths Needs of School Leavers Entering Employment, Symposium Proceedings,* Books 6, 11, 14.

JACKSON, P. H. and NOVICK, M. R. (1970). Maximising the validity of a unit-weight composite as a function of relative component lengths with a fixed total testing time. *Psychometrika,* Vol. 35, pp. 333–347.

JEFFERIES, P. M. (1978). *Mathematics in Nursing, 5th Edition.* London, Baillière Tindall.

JERNIGAN, D. K. (1980). Testing–A learning not a grading process. *Nursing Outlook,* Vol. 28, February, pp. 120–121.

JESSEE, R. W. and MCHENRY, R. W. (1975). *Self-Teaching Tests in Arithmetic for Nurses, 9th Edition.* St Louis, Mosby.

KEANE, C. B. and FLETCHER, S. M. (1980). *Drugs and Solutions, a Programmed Introduction, 4th Edition.* Philadelphia, W. B. Saunders Co.

KENNY, D. J. (1969). Drug administration errors. *The Hospital,* Vol. 65, February, pp. 55–57.

KERN, M. S. (1968). New ideas about drug systems. *American Journal of Nursing,* Vol. 68, pp. 1251–1253.

KEYWOOD, O. (1978). The hazards of orally administered drugs. *Nursing Mirror,* Vol. 1465, February, p. 41.

LAWLER, R. (1974). Mastery learning and remedial prescriptions in computer managed instruction. *Journal of Experimental Education,* Vol. 43, pp. 45–52.

LAYTON, J. (1975). Instructional packaging. *Journal of Nursing Education,* November, pp. 26–30.

LEEDS HOSPITAL. (1973). See Ford, P. M. and Ellis, S. 1973.

LEWIS, L. W. and LUVERNE WOLFF (1978). *Lippincott's State Board Exam Review for Nurses.* Philadelphia, J. B. Lippincott Co.

LINDSAY, C., MORRISON, J. and KELLEY, E. J. (1974). Professional obselescence: implications for professional education. *Adult Education,* Vol. 25, No. 1, pp. 3–22.

LINDSAY, M. (1980a). Lack of library services for nurses. *Nursing Times,* Vol. 76, January, p. 160.

LINDSAY, M. (1980b). Library service: shelving a learner's problems. *Nursing Mirror,* Vol. 151, July, No. 2, p. 30.

LINDSAY, R. L. (1980). *Mathematics and Engineering, 2nd Edition.* Engineering Industries Training Board.

LINN, R. L. and SLINDE, J. A. (1977). The determination of significance of change between pre- and post-testing periods. *Review of Educational Research,* Vol. 47, No. 1, pp. 121–150.

LIPPERT, H. and LEHMANN, H. P. (1978). *S.I. Units in Medicine.* Baltimore, Urban and Schwarzenberg.

LIPSEY, S. I. (1977). *Maths for Nursing Science: a programmed text, 2nd Edition.* New York, John Wiley.

LORD, F. M. (1967). A paradox in the interpretation of group comparisons. *Psychological Bulletin,* Vol. 68, No. 5, pp. 304–305.

LORD, F. M. (1969). Statistical adjustments when comparing pre-existing groups. *Psychological Bulletin,* Vol. 72, No. 5, pp. 336–337.

LOUGHLIN, T. M., SHIVELY, V. M., PECK, J. and DAVIS, E. (1964). A comparative study of supervised and unsupervised library periods for student nurses in psychiatric nursing. *Journal of Psychiatric Nursing,* pp. 345–9.

LUMSDEN, D. B. (1974). Another look at programmed instruction in nursing education. *International Nursing Review,* Vol. 21, November, p. 187, p. 183.

MARSHALL, J. C. and HALES, L. W. (1971). *Classroom Test Construction.* Massachusetts, Addison-Wesley.

MARSON, S. N. (1972). Programmed Instruction—panacea or passing gimmick? *International Nursing Review,* Vol. 19, March, pp. 126–137.

MARSON, S. N. (1975). What happened to programmed learning? *Nursing Times,* September, pp. 1425–1427.

MCCLAIN, M. E. (1966). *Simplified Arithmetic for Nurses, 3rd Edition.* Philadelphia, Saunders.

MCELROY, N. L., CARR, J. J. and CARR, B. L. (1977). *Simplified Maths for Nurses.* New York, Arco Publishing.

MCGEE, H. M. (1955). Measurement of authoritarianism and its relation to teachers' classroom behaviour. *Genetic Psychology Monographs,* Vol. 52, pp. 89–146.

MCHENRY, R. W. (1980). *Self-teaching Tests in Arithmetic for Nurses, 10th Edition.* St Louis, Mosby.

MEDICAL DEFENCE UNION, THE, (1981). *Annual Report,* London.

MEDICI, G. A. (1980). *Drug Dosage Calculations.* Englewood Cliffs, New Jersey, Prentice Hall.

MEDICO-PHARMACEUTICAL FORUM OF THE ROYAL SOCIETY OF MEDICINE (1980). Dangerous mistakes in drug administration. *Natnews,* Vol. 17, February, pp. 8–10.

METRICATION BOARD (1977). *How to Write Metric.* London, HMSO.

MOORES, B. and MOULT, A. (1979). Patterns of nurse activity. *Journal of Advanced Nursing,* Vol. 4, pp. 137–149.

MORTON, J. B. and MACBETH, W. A. A. G. (1977). Correlations between staff, peer and self-assessments of 4th year students in surgery. *Medical Education,* Vol. 11, pp. 167–170.

Mueller, D. J. (1976). Mastery learning: partly boon, partly boondoggle. *Teachers College Record,* Vol. 78, September, pp. 41–52.

Myco, F. (1980). Nursing research information: are nurse educators and practioners seeking it out? *Journal of Advanced Nursing,* Vol. 5, No. 6, pp. 637–646.

Nance, J. L. (1969). On the delegation of responsibility. *The Canadian Nurse,* Vol. 65, November, pp. 29–30.

National Physics Laboratory (1977). *S.I. The International System of Units, 3rd Edition.* (ed. Chester H. Page and Paul Vigoureux), London, HMSO.

Newton, M. and Newton, D. W. (1977). Guidelines for handling drug errors. *Nursing,* Vol. 7, September, pp. 62–68.

Novick, M. R., Lewis, C. and Jackson, P. H. (1973). The estimation of proportions in m groups. *Psychometrika,* Vol. 38, No. 1, pp. 19–46.

Oppenheim, A. N. (1966). *Questionnaire Design and Attitude Measurement.* London, Heinemann.

Olsen, L. J., Ablon, L. J., Giangrasso, A. P. and Siner, H. B. (1978). *Medical Dosage Calculations, 2nd Edition.* California, Benjamin/Cummings Publishing Co. Inc.

Osburn, H. G. (1968). Item sampling for achievement testing. *Educational and Psychological Measurement,* Vol. 28, pp. 95–104.

Oxford, R. H. A. (1974). Fatal confusion over child's drug dosage. *Nursing Mirror,* Vol. 139, August, p. 45.

Oxford, R. H. A. (1974). Measure for Measure—Inquiry into death of 3 year old given almost 17 times the proper dose of Nepenthe. *Nursing Times,* Vol. 70, August, p. 1258.

Palmer, D. A. (1980). Unit dose. *American Journal of Nursing,* Vol. 80, November, pp. 2062–3.

Perlstein, P. H., Callison, C., White, M., Barnes, B. and Neil, K. E. (1979). Errors in drug computations during newborn intensive care. *American Journal of Diseases of Children,* Vol. 133, No. 4, April, pp. 376–9.

Pickup, A. J. (1976). Aims, objectives and evaluations in vocational education. *Coombe Lodge Reports,* Vol. 9, No. 10, pp. 301–306.

Pirie, S. E. B. (1981) *Mathematics in Medicine.* Nottingham, Shell Centre for Mathematical Education.

Pirie, S. E. B. (1982). *Mathematics in the Ward—Drug Calculations.* Cheltenham, Stanley Thornes.

Polansky, N., Lippitt, R. and Redl, F. (1950). An investigation of behavioural contagion in groups. *Human Relations,* Vol. 3, pp. 319–348.

Popham, W. J. (1978). *Criterion-Referenced Measurement.* Englewood Cliffs, Prentice-Hall.

Popham, W. J. and Husek, T. R. (1969). Implications of criterion referenced measurement. *Journal of Educational Measurement,* Vol. 6, No. 1, pp. 1–9.

Price, G. G. (1963). *Self-study Guide of Maths used in Nursing.* New York, Putnam.

Richards, J. M. (1975). A stimulation study of the use of change measures to compare educational programs. *American Educational Research Journal,* Vol. 12, pp. 299–311.

Rosier, M. (1967). *Nursing Mathematics.* Oxford University Press.

RUSSELL, D. H. (1953). What does research say about self-evaluation? *Journal of Educational Research,* Vol. 66, No. 8, pp. 561–573.

SACKHEIM, G. I. and ROBINS, L. (1974). *Programmed Maths for Nurses, 3rd Edition.* Collier Macmillan.

SAXTON, D. F., ERCOLANO, N. H. and WALTER, J. F. (1977). *Programmed Instruction in Arithmetic, Doses and Solutions, 4th Edition.* St Louis, Mosby.

SCHOLES, M. and WIGMORE, H. (1967). Drug errors reduced. *Nursing Times,* April, pp. 563–4.

SCOTTISH HOME AND HEALTH DEPARTMENT (1967). (North Eastern Regional Hospital Board, Work Study Department). *Scottish Health Study No. 3: Nurses' work in hospitals in the N.E. Region.*

SHANKS, K. (1979). Warning: library useage may be habit forming. *Journal of Continuing Education in Nursing,* Vol. 10, No. 2, pp. 19–21.

SKARRATT, R. (1980). Student centred learning in nurse education. *Nursing Times,* Vol. 76, May, p. 953.

SKELLEY, E. G. (1971). *Medications and Maths for the Nurse and Instructor's Guide.* New York, Delmar.

SIEGEL, S. (1956). *Non-parametric Statistics for the Behavioural Sciences.* Kogakusha, Tokyo, McGraw-Hill.

SLOTNICKE, H. B. (1981). An approach to mathematical literacy for medical students. *Medical Education,* Vol. 15, January, pp. 11–16.

SMALL, M., ROMBERG, T. and CARNAHAN, R. (1979). *Teacher-Student Observation Procedures and the Training of Observers for Co-ordinated Study.* Madison, Wisconsin Research and Development Center, University of Wisconsin.

SPENCER, M. (1979). Did the students learn? Comparison of different study methods. *Nursing Times,* January, pp. 35–37.

STAKE, R. E. (1971). Testing hazards in performance contracting. *Phi Delta Kappan,* Vol. 52, June.

STEPHENSON, J. (1973). The use of nursing information (libraries). *Nursing Mirror,* August, pp. 46–47.

STEWART, D. Y., KELLY, J. and DINEL, B. A. (1976). Unit-dose medication; a nursing perspective. *American Journal of Nursing,* Vol. 76, pp. 1308–1310.

TABOR, R. B. (1979). Professional knowledge and the nurse. *Nursing Times,* November, pp. 1983–4.

TAYLOR, C. E. (1978). *Mathematics for Nursing.* Boston, Little Brown and Co.

TIDSKR SVER SJUKSKOT (1976a). Wrong injection of heparin. Vol. 43, No. 13, July, pp. 53–4.

TIDSKR SVER SJUKSKOT (1976b). Wrong drug dosage. Vol. 43, No. 18, October, p. 51.

VERE, D. W. (1965). Errors of complex prescribing. *Lancet,* Vol. 1, pp. 370–373.

WALSER, K. P. (1977). A college course for nurses on the utilisation of library resources. *Bulletin of Medical Library Association,* Vol. 56, No. 2, April, pp. 265–7.

WALTERS, S., BARKER, D. and WILKENS, C. (1979). Joint Nursing Pharmacy program helps reduce medication errors. *Hospital,* Vol. 53, March, pp. 141–4.

WARWICK HOSPITAL (1974). Safer drug handling (unit dose at Central Hospital, Warwick). *Nursing Mirror,* Vol. 139, September, p. 55.

WATCHORN, G. W. (1976). *Medical Calculations for Nurses, 2nd Edition.* Faber and Faber.

WEAVER, M. E. and KOEHLER, V. J. (1966). *Programmed Mathematics of Drugs and Solutions, 3rd Edition.* Philadelphia, Lippincott.

WILKINSON, P. W., NOBLE, T. C., GRAY, G. and SPENCE, O. (1973). Inaccuracies in measurement of dried milk powders. *British Medical Journal,* Vol. 2, pp. 15–17.

WILLIAMS, M. A. (1977). Quantification of direct nursing care activities. *Journal of Nursing Administration,* Vol. 7, October, pp. 15–18 and 49–51.

WILLIAMSON, K. C. and WHITE, S. J. (1974). Pharmacology competence ensured. *Hospitals,* J.A.H.A. Vol. 48, September, pp. 95–98.

WITTKOPF, B. (1972). Self-instruction for student learning. *American Journal of Nursing,* Vol. 72, pp. 2032–2034.

WOODBURY, M. A. and NOVICK, M. R. (1968). Maxismising the validity of a test battery as a function of relative test lengths for a fixed total testing time. *Journal of Mathematical Psychology,* Vol. 5, pp. 242–259.

WORLD HEALTH ORGANISATION (1978). Competency-based curriculum development in medical education. *Public Health Paper No. 68.*

WRIGHTSTONE, J. W. (1951). Measuring the social climate of a classroom. *Journal of Educational Research,* Vol. 44, pp. 341–351.

WYMAN, J. and FERNAU, K. (1977). Developing a criterion-referenced tool. *Nursing Outlook,* Vol. 25, pp. 584–6.

YUNEK, M. (1980). Self-assessment of learning needs. *Journal of Continuing Education in Nursing,* Vol. 11, September, No. 5, pp. 36–41.

Nurses and Mathematics

Deficiencies in Basic Mat[illegible]
Development and Evalu[illegible] Methods [illegible] and
Treatment

SUSAN PIRIE
M.A., Ph.D.

AIMS OF THE SERIES

To encourage the appreciation and dissemination of nursing research by making relevant studies of high quality available to the profession at reasonable cost.

The RCN is very happy indeed to publish this series of research reports. The projects were chosen by the individual research worker and the findings are those of the researcher and relate to the particular subject in the situation in which it was studied. The RCN in accordance with its policy of promoting research awareness among members of the profession commends this series for study but views expressed do not necessarily reflect RCN policy.

ISBN 0-902606-92-1

British Library Cataloguing in Publication Data

Published by
The Royal College of Nursing
of the United Kingdom,
Cavendish Square, London, W1M 0AB.

Printed by The Whitefriars